Dedicated to my family:

brother George; sister, Marion;

husband, Gene Sr.; son, Gene Jr.; daughter, Ladonna;

son-in-law, Steve; and granddaughter, Chrissie.

ACKNOWLEDGMENTS

My support van drivers: Edna, Blanche, Cecilia, Gene, and Ladonna. You've given me enough love and caring to fill a lifetime! On an adventure like this, it takes a certain kind of person to be able to handle the emergencies and time frames and keep a level head in all types of circumstances.

Judy Rogers, who was my "book doctor."

Virginia Steinwig, who labeled most of the pictures and helped in so many other ways.

Dorothy Patchett Eby, a special friend who was always there to help.

Steve Upton and his family from Whirlpool; Ellsworth McKee from McKee Baking Company; and my brother, George Patterson, who gave financial assistance that helped to make the trip possible.

. . . and scores of people around the world who helped in some way to move me toward the finish line!

4,200 MILES
Across Canada
Summer 1993

1,000 MILES
British Columbia
Summer 1988

2,500 MILES
Across America
Spring 1987

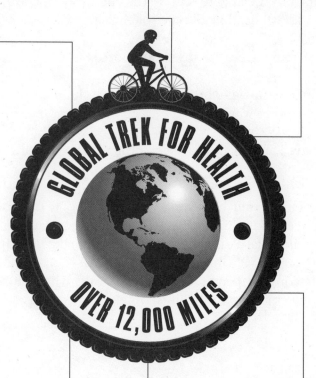

2,000 MILES
Asian Countries
Spring 1988

1,800 MILES
Europe
Fall 1987

600 MILES
Brisbane-Sydney
Fall 1992

CONTENTS

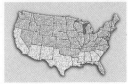
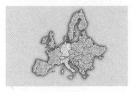
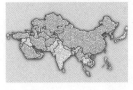

CONTENTS *continued*

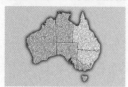
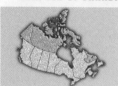

INTRODUCTION

For many years I taught health education classes. I know that, with few exceptions, we can restore men and women to health. One day I began to wonder what just one person could do to encourage thousands of people to seek a lifestyle that would bring true fulfillment to their lives. The answer, I decided, was to demonstrate the benefits of a healthy lifestyle.

So in 1987, at the age of 68, I began a trek that would take me around the world on a bicycle, finishing my journey at the age of 75. I rode 50 to 80 miles a day in temperatures ranging from 34° to 110°F. Through every kind of weather, on every kind of road, through gorgeous countryside and untamed wilderness, I rode. I am now convinced our bodies are capable of performing far beyond what we have asked of them.

Some people wake up in the morning with a heart bursting with gratitude for the chance to live another day. For others life has become a drudgery; happiness seems to have drifted away with time. Headaches, sore joints, and clogged arteries begin to require more and more pills until little remains of a once-buoyant spirit. Is there anything we can do to pick up the broken pieces and put them together again?

Yes!

Ten steps, carefully followed, will change—wonderfully change—any situation, no matter how impossible it may seem. These steps are the keys to health and happiness. The closer we harmonize with nature, the better we feel and the longer we will live. Think of it as a **FRESH START**:

Fresh air	**S**unshine
Rest	**T**he use of water
Exercise	**A**bstemiousness
Simple diet	**R**estoration
Happiness	**T**rust in divine power

Now come with me to the far corners of the globe where adventure, drama, danger, miracles, and much more await!

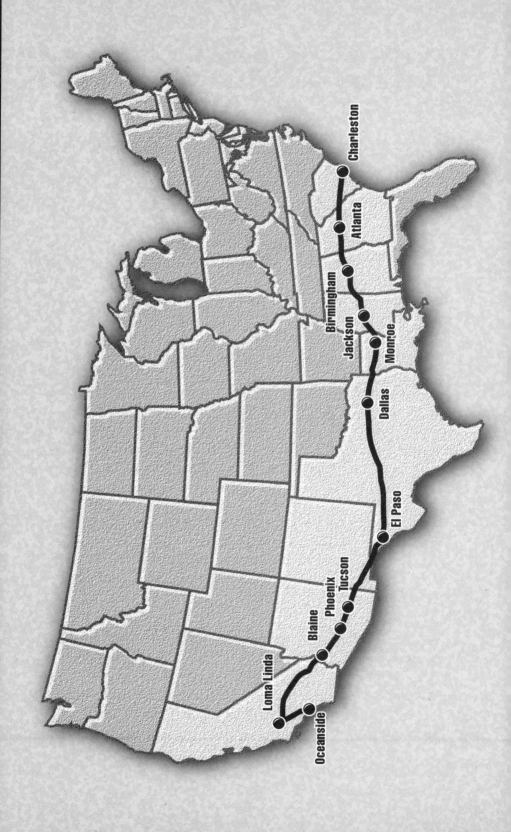

ACROSS AMERICA

Charleston

Atlanta

Birmingham

Jackson

Monroe

Dallas

El Paso

Tucson

Phoenix

Blaine

Loma Linda

Oceanside

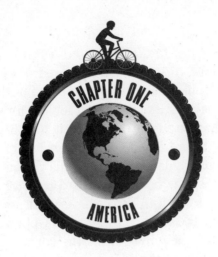

CHAPTER ONE

AMERICA

PREPARATION

I hugged my husband and my son, Gene Sr. and Gene Jr., good-bye and promised to be careful, then climbed into the driver's seat of my 21-foot Mini-Cruiser. The rack on the back of the van held my brand-new bicycle, a gift from a FRESH START for Health program client. A last look in the rearview mirror revealed the two of them standing together, with looks of amazement and concern chasing across their faces, as I pulled out of the driveway of our Berrien Springs, Michigan, home. Patches of snow still crowded into shady areas of the yard.

It was February 17, 1987, and I was a woman with a mission. At the age of 68 I planned to cross the United States on a bicycle. My mission? To show that we should be able to do the things we want to do. At any age. I wanted everybody to feel as good as I did, to feel better and live longer, to know that health is a gift. I hoped my trip would encourage others to learn about—and to live—healthier lifestyles.

In spite of my excitement, questions surfaced in my mind. Would I have the endurance to climb over the mountains, ride through the storms, and cover the necessary miles as I crossed the continent? Could I do it in two months as I had planned? What dangers lurked out there to hinder me from reaching my goal? Was I really sure about all this? A hundred butterflies fluttered across the pit of my stomach. My foot pressed a little harder on the gas pedal, and the Mini-Cruiser picked up speed. I was on my way!

I had selected California's Capistrano Beach as the official starting point for my journey. As I drove west I looked forward to overnight visits with friends along the way. I spent that first evening at the home of Dr. Demil and Edna Andreassen in O'Fallion, Missouri, friends from our college days at Walla Walla College. Edna and I had both become nurses. She had volunteered to drive the Mini-Cruiser and accompany me for at least three weeks of the journey.

We breakfasted the next morning on raspberries, whole-wheat toast, and granola. I knew that eating the correct foods was important to my performance. Demil wished me good luck, then Edna and I were on our way.

On February 24 we arrived in Escondido, California, where my brother George and sister, Marion, both widowed, shared a winter home. Their warm welcome couldn't hide their concern about my plans, however. George tried to discourage what he viewed as his older sister's "foolishness." When they finally realized that this was something I needed to do, they joined in the spirit of the venture as we made final arrangements for takeoff.

We decided to change the starting point from Highway 74 at Capistrano Beach to Highway 76 in Oceanside. The cliffs on Highway 74 came straight down to the edge of the road, leaving no space for a shoulder and posing risk to a cyclist.

We took my bike to a local shop to have it checked over. "We may have to put on a new chain," announced the young attendant at the shop, as he looked at the bike.

George and I stared at him in amazement. "A new chain! Why, I've hardly ridden the bike yet!"

Jim, the manager, came out to take a look. "Looks pretty messed up to me," he remarked.

I envisioned a $40 charge for an overhaul and decided to plead my case. "Look, the bike was new when I put it on the rack," I explained. "I just left Michigan a week ago, and traveled on freeways covered with ice, snow, salt, and sand, and it does look as if most of it got on the bike. But I'm going to ride this bicycle across

America with a friend driving a support van. I just need to be sure the bike's ready to go."

They agreed to check everything out for me. "I can set up a plan for bicycle clubs to escort you along your route," Jim suggested as he worked. "They could ride with you to the next agreed-on point."

I considered his offer. How much time might this attention cost me? How many times might I have to wait for a club to meet me? What if the press delayed me, the weather was bad, or if I took a wrong turn? Regretfully, I decided to decline. "Thanks, Jim, but by the time it was all organized I could be almost through Arizona. I don't want to delay the trip."

He stared at me in astonishment. "Do you mean to tell me that you're going across these United States alone? You'll never make it!"

When my bombardier stopped for a breath I quickly counterattacked. (After all, who was going to stand up for me out there on the road? I might as well start practicing now.) "Of course, I'll make it! I ran a live-in conditioning center until the day before I left Michigan. Now I'm doing my best to be ready to leave Oceanside by next Monday."

We stared at each other across the muddy bicycle, then Jim grinned and shook his head. I think we had both enjoyed the exchange.

We returned for the bike the next day. It shone like new, with everything cleaned, carefully checked, and oiled. "No charge!" Jim smiled.

Looking back, I wouldn't blame anyone for being of the same mind as the young man at the bicycle shop. Certainly my white hair and my age could throw people who hadn't seen me in action. (When I was in my 60s, I clocked 8.6 seconds in the 50-meter track event in the Senior Olympics.) One of five children growing up on a farm in Canada, I had ridden horses and bicycles, ice-skated, climbed mountains, and swum in lakes. My love of the outdoors has continued throughout my life.

My simple diet is another reason for my abounding energy, day after day. My daily menu includes lentils or other legumes or vegetables, potato dishes, whole-wheat bread, whole-grain cereals, fresh salads, and fruits. These foods release stored glycogen more slowly than energy from candy bars and other refined foods. I don't use soft drinks, and drink only water between meals.

One last obligation remained before I started my trip. I had accepted an invitation to speak at UPDATE, the annual School of Public Health convention held at Loma Linda University, just a few miles north of Oceanside.

As I waited to speak, I remembered the excitement of a night 47 years before when I had stood on this same platform to receive my nurse's cap, the symbol of my status as a "real" student nurse. I recalled the words of the Nightingale pledge: "I solemnly pledge myself before God and in the presence of this assembly . . . to pass my life in purity . . . I will not take or knowingly administer any harmful drug . . . I will endeavor to aid the physician in his work . . ."

Hearing my name, I was jarred back to the present. "Charlotte Hamlin graduated from the School of Nursing in 1943, and from the School of Public Health in 1972, where she earned a master's degree in Public Health Nutrition and Health Education. Two days from now," the speaker continued, "she plans to begin a 2,500-mile walk and bicycle ride across America to promote longer life through better living."

I looked out over the gathering of physicians, dentists, nurses, environmentalists, and other allied health personnel scattered through the audience. Could I convey to them how strongly I believed in my mission? I took a deep breath and stepped to the podium.

"We have a solemn responsibility to present the harmonious development of body, mind, and soul to the world. Today new inventions, expensive equipment, and a medicine for every symptom are at our disposal. Even so, heart disease and cancer are epidemic in our country. Diabetes and other degenerative diseases are taking their toll, while great populations in China and Southeastern Asia seldom see a heart attack, and the funds used for medical care are minimal in comparison to Western countries."

As I continued to speak I looked at the faces of the audience. *Were they really hearing me?* I wondered.

"Our bodies are living temples in which the Spirit of God dwells. Sometimes we tend to forget how really valuable we are. I think of the Temple of the Dawn in Bangkok. Rising almost straight up into the blue sky, it takes your breath away. Some who worship there spend much of their lives cementing beautiful patterns from broken pieces of pottery on the outside walls. As the sun shines on them, they sparkle like millions of diamonds. No sacrifice is too great for their gods. Can we offer less?

"It is my plan to implement the FRESH START principles of health into my upcoming adventure. Pray that I will be an example out there on the road, encouraging others to feel more responsible for their own health and, in turn, passing on their good fortune to those around them. After all, happiness and even restoration to health are in the FRESH START formula, and are the result of following these health principles."

Suddenly I was eager to get on the road.

ON THE WAY

I waded into the water at the edge of the Pacific Ocean, the official beginning of my journey across the United States. George and Marion were there for the occasion, as well as a niece and her children. So was Dottie, my roommate from college days. Short and blond, always looking for a way to help someone, Dottie reminded me of a firefly—never landing, but lighting the way as she goes. She had lent me a camera, tapes, and a tape recorder for the trip.

Afterward Marion and I walked together through Oceanside. We reminisced about the past and about some of our plans for the future. We shared memories of happy times we'd had with our late sister, Ruth. Identical twins, Marion and Ruth had trained together for nursing careers. Ruth's death had been a great loss to all of us, but hardest of all for Marion. We had walked more than four miles before we joined George and Edna for lunch in a little cafe. After eating, we quickly said goodbye. It was easier that way.

Feelings of excitement rippled through me as I mounted my bicycle. I pushed down on the pedals and the bicycle began to roll forward. I was on my way! Edna, driving the support van, would start out a little later, pass me, and park by the side of the road. If I needed anything I'd stop at the van. Otherwise, on I'd go!

I met with a steep grade for about six miles on Highway 395 and had to walk some of the way, pushing 38 pounds of bicycle, including a small handlebar bag. Happily for me, I had lots of energy, no sore muscles, and felt ready to burst at the seams with gratitude and confidence that everything was going to be all right.

Twenty-one miles the first afternoon, walking and riding, wasn't a bad beginning. We spent the night behind a service station. Although a little noisy, it was better than parking out on the open road. (We made it a practice to always park close enough to civilization so that someone could hear the emergency whistle I wore around my neck.)

The next morning we returned to where I had stopped the evening before. As on the previous afternoon, I rode from gently rolling hills to vast, irrigated citrus groves and vineyards, broken up by valleys and green trees. At first I didn't do much sightseeing as I rode along, but concentrated on the highway before me. I was afraid that if I allowed my attention to wander I might go head over heels down a steep hill or end up in a ditch.

I started out on the alternate route near the freeway, a small washboard of a road, and somehow ended up on the freeway. It was delightful! I could really sail along, except for those places where construction was in progress and a great chasm left me little room for pedaling. Several patrol cars passed me on the freeway, but none of them stopped.

This is great! I thought. *Maybe they'll let this poor old soul stay on the freeway all the way to Charleston, South Carolina!*

Before I knew it, I had gone all the way to Corona instead of taking Highway 215 to Loma Linda, where we were to stay with Dottie overnight. I'd lost Edna and could only hope she'd find me. I called Dorothy, who came and picked me up. Miraculously, just as Edna decided to stop at a service station for directions, we spotted the van among those thousands of cars whizzing along in the dusk and escorted her in. In view of several delays along the way I decided 53 miles for the day wasn't bad. (I also decided it would take a couple weeks on the road to completely toughen up, especially the place where I sit. Nothing but time changes *that* flesh into leather!)

BATTLING A DESERT STORM

I had developed an inflammation in my right eye. If the hot sun and dust were to irritate it trouble could follow. Dorothy's son, Tim, an ophthalmologist at Loma Linda Medical Center, examined it before we left the next day. Fortunately, some drops Edna had with her were all we needed to clear up the inflammation. We picked up some supplies and were on our way again.

From the beginning of my trip I was very particular about starting where I had stopped the day before. Corona, my starting point of the day, was far west of where I should have been. Since I could have gone northeast on Highway 79 and made it to Banning the night before, saving about 15 miles, I decided to leave from Loma Linda, about an equal distance. I put on my helmet and headed across the Timoteo Canyon Road. Edna and I planned to meet in Banning, where we would park for the night at Dr. Charles Thomas's health conditioning center.

Dr. Thomas, who had been one of my professors at Loma Linda University years before, had changed the course of the disease for numerous people who suffered from arthritis, back problems, injuries, depression, and other ailments. He felt that treatment of the affliction by strengthening the immune system and improving the mental outlook would produce more lasting results. The center used hot and cold packs, massage, diathermy, daily workouts on indoor equipment or outdoor walking, and a healthy diet to treat the patients.

As I rode across the bumpy road that ran over the dry, almost uninhabited desert, I realized that mountains hemmed me in on all sides. A strong head wind from the east began to whistle through the canyon toward me, and black storm clouds boiled against each other overhead. As I struggled against the force of the elements I wondered if this was why so few dwellings dotted the countryside.

Finally, I came upon a fairly new building sitting alone in the desert. After parking my bike I went inside to call the center. I asked the secretary to tell Edna I would be arriving late due to the weather. As I turned to leave, a young man, who had overheard my conversation, introduced himself as Bill and offered me a ride to Banning. I thanked him, but since he didn't plan to leave for several hours I decided to continue on my way alone.

Back on the highway, I rode through a gathering storm. A middle-aged man in a pickup truck going in the opposite direction stopped to ask if I would like a ride. He stared at the ACROSS AMERICA banner around my waist.

"I must ride my bicycle all the way," I told him. "But thanks anyway."

I bumped along the road for another hour. The storm was still brewing but hadn't boiled over yet. Then the man in the pickup stopped again. Although I felt uneasy out there alone with so few cars passing by, I sensed I shouldn't accept his offer. "Thanks anyway," I said again, "but I'll just keep riding."

He left, and I didn't see him again.

Finally, the pedals refused to take me any farther in the fierce gale. I got off and began pushing my bicycle along the road. Thunder and lightning flashed and huge drops of rain blew in my face. The ever-blackening clouds hid the sun, but its rays created a gold frame around the edges of the clouds. Less than three days on the road and here I was helpless in the clutches of a storm. Had this whole thing been a mistake?

No! I pushed the question from my mind. Not once on the long trek would I allow myself to cling to such thoughts or to consider giving up. "God, I need help," I whispered. I continued walking, and soon I heard the sound of a motor. The young man who had offered me a ride when I stopped to use the phone pulled up beside me. He laid my bicycle in the back of his pickup and I climbed into the cab, sheltered from the storm. I took careful note of the landscape and all possible identification marks so that Edna could bring me back in the morning to start the next day's ride.

Someone might ask, "Weren't you foolish to have a support van and not have it there with you?"

Yes, and no. Usually the support driver passed me, then stopped and waited farther down the road, depending on the need. If the van stayed close to me, whether ahead or behind, it would cut down on my visibility. The slow speed would also be very hard on the van's motor.

When I had left at 2:00, it had been a beautiful day and Banning wasn't far away. Since Edna hadn't finished her shopping, it seemed simpler for her just to skip over to Banning on the freeway. And in this particular situation it might have been more dangerous for Edna had she been with me. On my trip to California from Michigan a garage attendant in Indio, California, told me he had personally seen five campers blown over in strong winds. If this had happened to Edna and the Mini-Cruiser it would have been the end of our trek.

Bill dropped me off in Banning. I wondered if he realized that God knew I'd need him to answer my prayer. By the time I found the center, darkness filled the sky and a soft drizzle was all that remained of the angry weather. A very relieved Edna welcomed me. Before going to bed we enjoyed a relaxing soak in the Jacuzzi. I had covered only 13 miles, but I probably had used more energy than in all the miles I had covered the previous day.

ON THE INTERSTATE—BUT FOR HOW LONG?

The next morning we returned to the point where I had stopped the evening before. Although overcast and cool, the weather was pleasant and windless. I waved goodbye to Edna as she pulled ahead of me in the van.

A flood of memories filled my thoughts as I rode. San Bernardino, a little farther north, is the gateway to Lake Arrowhead, Big Bear Lake, and other mountain resorts. As a student nurse nearly 50 years before, I had climbed in those mountains and slept under the stars. Once I even swam across Lake Arrowhead without a boat to accompany me. To my right lay San

Jacinto. I had climbed to the top when I was a young assistant camp nurse for 70 boys and counselors. So I enjoyed adventure long before I started on this latest journey.

The miles flew by. I passed near Beaumont and Banning, where I had held cooking schools while in graduate school. *Time to stop dreaming,* I told myself. Here I was on Interstate 10, one of the famous arteries of travel across the United States, riding down the shoulder of the freeway on a bicycle! I knew that bicycles were off limits here, but somehow I had a feeling that this was where I belonged. I prayed, "Please give me the words to speak when the California highway patrolman pulls up behind me (as he surely will, sooner or later). Thank You for keeping me safe. Amen."

On the other side of the mountain, farther north on SR 38, lay Barton Flats. One summer another student and I had spent a month at the campsite of Dr. and Mrs. Crooks. At the time, Dr. Crooks was the anatomy teacher at Loma Linda University, and a very good one. Due to poor eating habits his wife, Hulda, a dietitian, had suffered health problems when younger. Dr. Crooks wisely found ways to keep her outdoors and active in the fresh air and sunshine. She has remained busy and in good health. In fact, since the age of 81 she has climbed 86 of the 268 officially registered mountains of southern California, including numerous climbs on Mt. Whitney. The body's performance during our time on earth "is largely dependent on the intelligent care we give to it," she says.

My eyes scanned the horizon. Directly north of Banning, beyond the foothills, are the highest mountains in southern California, including San Gorgonio (11,502 feet). I had climbed that mountain twice half a century earlier. I wondered if I could make it to the top now if I tried.

About noon the wind picked up. Carl Love from Riverside's *Press Enterprise* met me as he traveled west. When he saw my ACROSS AMERICA sign he turned around and came back to interview me and take pictures for an article for the next day's newspaper. The media proved to be my most successful means of spreading the good news of health.

"I don't think you're living too healthfully by being on the interstate," he observed. He was probably right, but since I was alone most of the time it was still the best place for me to be.

Underway once more, I scooted down and through Palm Springs, dodging in and out of the heavy traffic. What a paradise! There was so much to see, but I knew I mustn't lose sight of my goal. I crossed Bob Hope Drive, rode across the overpass above the interstate, and was once more riding with the wind. A car horn sounded nearby. Looking toward the median, I saw a man standing beside his car exposing himself. Summoning all available energy, I pedaled up the hill in front of me, but it felt as though I was barely crawling. Thankfully, he didn't try to follow me.

Friday and Saturday nights we stayed at Tamarisk RV Park in Desert Center. Saturday was my day to rest. Edna and I enjoyed walking into the desert, away from the flying traffic. We discovered that a couple at the park, Noreen and Harold Prosch, had been classmates of Edna's during nursing school.

On Sunday we crossed over the Colorado River into Arizona. How thankful we were that California was behind us and we were both doing well, ready for the next segment of our trip. Our pleasure increased at the sight of lupines and other flowers that lifted their colorful faces in large patches of blues and yellows. We spent the night at Central Arizona Project Canal.

Monday morning I had ridden only two-and-one-half miles, when there he was—every crease on his pressed uniform in the right place, every button shining, and his badge dazzling in the rays of the sun. The Arizona State Patrol! He listened silently as I pled my case. I told him about my transcontinental trek and how I hoped it would make older people more aware of their potential. I mentioned the importance of senior citizens contributing to society instead of being a drain on the younger generation.

He seemed willing to keep listening, so I forged ahead. I told him of my concern about alternate routes with narrow roads (often without shoulders) and, frequently, no place for Edna to park the van. I mentioned the long stretches with little or no traffic and my concern about being out there alone.

"I know you're right," he said finally. "Just be careful, please. There's really no place that is safe out here."

"I cannot thank you enough," I said, fervently shaking his hand. "I'm encouraged by your kindness. I want to do my best and be a good example when I speak in schools, hospitals, churches—and even out here on the road." From that day on, perhaps through some state patrol grapevine, they seemed to know when I was coming through.

Blessings had showered us all along the way that first week on the road. I decided to list them. I was thankful:

1. For Edna—her healthy meals, good timing, good nature, and concern for my safety.

2. That the man in the median hadn't followed me.

3. For those times when I had had a tail wind as the bike and I climbed hills.

4. That we were in Arizona.

5. That we had found satisfactory places to stop every night.

6. That I was allowed to travel on the freeway shoulder (so far).

7. That I was rolling along!

LOST!

The weather was cool, the road fairly smooth, and the people wonderful. But, oh, my gluteus maximus! By March 10 the part of my body that sat on the bike seat for hours began to complain. Putting a hot water bottle on the seat didn't work. The water just settled where I wasn't. In fact, the bottle itself refused to stay in place. As I rode along feeling sorry for myself, I found a cute little teddy bear at the side of the road. He was soft and clean and cooperated much better than the hot water bottle.

Soon we were in the gentle, rolling hills of desert countryside. Several varieties of cacti and other flora helped take my mind off the road. The only animals I saw as I traveled the freeway were dead ones that provided dinner for the vultures.

One night we camped beside a building at Buckeye Municipal Airport. Russ Adams, the owner of the airport, had flown B-26s in

TO YOUR HEALTH!

In the introduction I mentioned the FRESH START for Health program. As we cross the Colorado River into Arizona, let's refer to the first of those principles of health represented by the acronym FRESH START.

The "F" stands for Fresh air. *Lack of oxygen can lead to tissue death and disease conditions, such as heart attacks, strokes, arthritis, and even cancer. Fresh outdoor air carries negative ions; stale indoor air has more positive ions. These positive ions contribute to allergy symptoms, headaches, and irritability. Negative ions help to produce a tranquil, comfortable feeling and exhilaration.*

Dr. George Chen, author of Air-Pressure, Gift of Heaven, *writes that air pollution and smog decrease the amount of negative ions in the air we breathe. The earth is naturally negatively charged from sunshine, or from the breakup of water droplets. That's probably why one feels better when near a waterfall, lake, or ocean. To have good health we need to breathe properly. Full, deep inhalations of pure air fill the lungs with oxygen and purify the blood. Try breathing in as deeply as you can from your diaphragm, not your chest, then let it out slowly through your mouth. Cough a couple times to get the stale residue air out of the bottom of your lungs. Each day take at least ten of these deep breaths while you're exercising.*

One of the better-known stories about the effects of fresh air concerns F. O. Stanley, inventor of the Stanley Steamer automobile. Given only a few months to live, he and his wife moved to Colorado, where he lived an additional 37 years before dying at age 93. Credit for his improved health went to the dry air in the high altitude, proper rest, and exercise.

Try to follow these guidelines:

1. *Practice deep breathing until it "clicks in" automatically.*
2. *Exercise to help keep the blood vessels open, thus allowing the red cells to carry more oxygen.*
3. *Air out your house daily and sleep with your windows open.*
4. *Green plants absorb carbon dioxide from the air and give off oxygen. Keep some in the house.*
5. *Spend as much time outdoors as possible.*

World War II. He had spent 12 years building a plane, carving the wooden ribs and covering the frame with fiber, and flying it for the first time in February 1986.

Now that's exciting! I thought. All I could take credit for was 58 miles of lifting my knees up and putting them back down again. But every day brought a new adventure. As we entered Phoenix (population 700,000), Edna and I lost track of each other. I headed for 19th and Van Buren streets, where I expected to meet her, but there was no Edna. I notified police headquarters that I had lost my support van, then waited. Four hours later our calls and the police calls meshed. Edna had understood that I would meet her at the highway patrol station on 23rd and Encento streets. We have no idea how we got our wires crossed. And I'd just as soon leave it a mystery—that way I have one chance out of two that *I* was right!

We stayed overnight across from the highway patrol office. It was March 11, and I had ridden 399 miles since leaving the afternoon of March 2. Not bad!

Sunday's weather turned quite cool, blustery, and rainy. Edna pulled the van off more often to wait for me. Rain soaked me in no time, and I had to stop and change clothes. My lined sail jacket had a rubberized surface and a hood that fit under my helmet, and was long enough to keep the rain off behind. It was dangerous to ride in heavy rain, though. The cars splashed me, the rearview mirror and my glasses fogged up, the road could be slippery, and I was miserable. It usually paid to wait out bad weather.

Texas Canyon Summit, with an altitude of 4,975 feet, lay ahead. To get over the top I would have to cross high chaparral country on a long, gradual grade. On the road over Snow Ridge a man stopped to check on me, concerned that the weather might maroon me there all night.

"Oh, no, I'll be all right," I answered with assurance.

Some time later he appeared again. He had gone 10 miles down the road, then turned around and come back. "I couldn't get you out of my mind, alone out here on the road with sleet on the ground and the cold of night coming on."

At that moment Edna drove up and stopped behind me. "Ah, here's my support van," I told him.

"You're all right, then?"

I assured him we would be fine, thanked him for stopping, and he went on his way. I wish now that I had gotten his name and address and sent him a thank-you note. It meant so much to me to remember all those extra miles he traveled just for me!

A good noon meal, a little siesta, and I headed east once more. I decided to make a quick telephone call home at a rest stop beside the road. I didn't want to miss Edna while I was off the road, though. She would soon be heading my way, and if she didn't see me she could be miles ahead of me in a few minutes, thinking *I* was still ahead of *her*. I called out to a trucker who was just getting ready to pull out of the rest area. "If you see a white-and-blue Mini-Cruiser with an ACROSS AMERICA sign in the window, would you please tell the driver that I'm behind her and on my way?"

I learned later that when he and a buddy in another semi spotted Edna, one of them pulled in front of her and the other behind. All three of them had a great visit, and the truckers enjoyed hearing about our trip and its purpose.

Small western towns dotted the countryside. Wide-open spaces gave me a feeling of freedom and relaxation. Cacti, sand, and more sand dominated the rolling hills as far as I could see. We stayed overnight in the parking lot of the hospital in Willcox, where the evening shift gave us a royal welcome. Edna had made some makeshift masks for me to wear to filter out the exhaust fumes. When I asked about buying several surgical masks (that I felt might be more efficient), the nurses gave me six.

The *Arizona Range* newspaper editor interviewed us the next morning and took pictures to run in the next day's paper. Then we were on our way again.

Some snow still remained on the higher peaks, and the weather on the plains was nippy. In the hills around Willcox, orchards, vineyards, and cotton fields replaced cattle ranches. In the early days these hills had harbored nearly as many fugitive gunslingers as cattle. Some of the smaller towns, like Pearce, were almost ghost towns, with boarded up windows and doors.

Suddenly we were over the border and into New Mexico, the third state on our itinerary. This was cotton country! And grape vineyards also began to dot the countryside. I rode by apple orchards. Snow covered the mountain peaks in the distance. What a picture! How thankful I felt to be alive in this great country of ours.

You haven't heard me say much about aches and pains or

exhaustion. The reason is that I didn't have any once the tired, sore bottom parts toughened up. Any other discomforts were minor and short-lived.

TO YOUR HEALTH!

As we cross the border from Arizona into New Mexico, let's take a minute and talk about the "R" in FRESH START, which stands for Rest.

Research shows that physical healing takes place faster during sleep. Many biochemical, physiological, and psychological events occur as we sleep. Most researchers believe a metabolic build-up occurs in the body during sleep—repairing, restoring, and preparing for the next day.

Sleep is preventive medicine. During sleep our body produces the protective substances in our bone marrow and lymph nodes that help fight off infection in greater amounts. Skin cells divide twice as fast, and the human growth hormone reaches its peak during the deep stages of sleep.

A nine-year study done by Drs. Breslow and Belloc, with about 7,000 subjects, indicates that a person needs seven to eight hours of sleep. The study also shows that too much or too little sleep seems to shorten our life span.

Americans spend an ever-increasing amount of money on sleeping medications. Much of the cost is a tragic waste. Sleeping pills disturb the REM, or deep sleep pattern, and the user often wakes up feeling tired and listless.

When teaching my students, I used Ministry of Healing, a textbook written by Ellen White, a proven authority on health. White says that God has given us a certain amount of "vital force." If we carefully preserve this life force the result is health. If we use this force too quickly the nervous system borrows power for the present from its resources of strength. In an effort to correct the condition a fever and other forms of illness can result.

Sometimes I wake up in the night, but why worry? Instead, I think of something pleasant, repeat Bible promises, or see how many different kinds of warblers I can remember. And there are many folks who would appreciate a little prayer on their behalf. I'm usually asleep before I get to the second name on the list!

If you have trouble sleeping, some of these ideas might help: exercise more, have a fixed time for going to bed, avoid late meals, avoid stimulants, practice deep breathing, sleep in a cool, quiet room with the window open, or relax one part of the body at a time. I'm feeling sleepy just thinking about it!

At Lordsburg we enjoyed a fresh salad—and pizza, a rare indulgence. I've found that simply-prepared foods, in as natural a form as possible, take less energy to digest and give better performance on the road.

The land became a great, flat plain between Lordsburg and Deming. The level ground was a rare treat. I maintained a speed of 12 to 14 miles per hour and didn't have to constantly change gears. With a lighter bike and more effort I could have increased the miles covered, but I had a long way to go and needed to pace myself.

About an hour down the road I stopped to take off a layer of clothes. If the van was near I could leave the extra clothes in it. Otherwise, I secured them on the rack behind me. In future travels in other countries when I didn't have a support vehicle, the bike bulged with sometimes as many as two to four panniers. The best advice I can give anyone: do not have one ounce more than is essential on either the bike or support vehicle. Too bad our traveling days were almost over before this lesson finally sank in!

Later that day a police officer stopped me to tell me what I already knew: I wasn't supposed to ride on the interstate. As I crossed the border into each state, one or two of these gentlemen usually pulled up behind me. Once we had the opportunity to talk things over and I was back on the road they must have passed the word along my route, because I was seldom stopped more than once in the same state. I really appreciated their understanding and had no fear of the flashing lights that periodically pulled up behind me. I'll always respect their courage in being out where danger is often not far away.

After hours of open plains, sagebrush, sand, and tumbleweeds, I completed my trek over the Continental Divide, a gradual upgrade to about 4,500 feet. New Mexico's state flower, the yucca, began to break the monotony of the landscape. Near the little town of Deming, fields of cotton and grain thrived on the water from the subsurface flow of the Mimbres River, a river that vanishes into the earth north of the city, then reappears down in Mexico.

I had been on the road for more than two weeks. I decided that if I ever had a flat tire Edna would take the bike to a shop or service station, and I would continue the trip by walking until she returned. That very morning I had a strong impression I should stop and pick up tire repair equipment. So we bought a pump, gauge, and tire patches at a bike shop. (I already had a new tire and tube in the van.) That afternoon Edna found me "out there," pushing my bike, the back tire flat from a nail. Off she went to have it repaired while I walked on. It felt absolutely wonderful to get off that seat and feel the surge of blood returning from my lower limbs, past the point where the pressure bore down under my thighs. Walking every day for a change of pace, mostly up hills, helped make the trek more interesting.

I chalked up seven miles before Edna returned with news. No one, including the truckers, knew how to change the tire! So she set off again on the interstate, where she spotted a young hitchhiker. Although naturally hesitant about stopping, she decided to take a chance. "Can you change a bike tire?" Edna asked the tall, blond young man.

"Sure," he answered. Rick Bunch, on his way to Dallas, proved every inch the gentleman. He turned the bicycle upside down on the interstate and went to work, using the items we'd bought that morning. In defense of common sense, all of us should learn how to change a tire on a car or bicycle. When I traveled alone on future trips I did have directions with me for changing a tire, but never once did I have to use them. Every day seemed to bring its own miracle. My tires always chose to go flat in the right places!

After supper I felt really chipper and it was cool out, so I decided to ride for a bit. "I'll take Rick on to Truck Stop 6," Edna said. "Maybe he can get a ride with a trucker."

"I'll meet you there," I promised, and started on my way. With the wind at my back and a good shoulder to travel on, I was flying low—so low that I missed the off-ramp. Darkness began to settle in. Since I didn't usually travel at night, the bike didn't have a light. Soon it was completely black, and I couldn't see well enough to continue, but neither could I just stand there in the dark. I began thinking about the "Man Wanted" flyer I'd seen posted in every truck stop in the area. This fugitive had stolen a semi and taken a woman and her 9-year-old daughter into the desert. When they refused to cooperate with his wishes, he shot them. They both lived, but the man was still at large.

Suddenly, directly in front of me, a police car pulled a car off onto the shoulder. Two state troopers, guns pulled, slowly made their way toward the car. I cautiously walked up to the open door of the patrol car and stood there by my bike until the officers returned. When I announced "I think I'm lost," both officers jumped. Neither had seen me in the dark. I realized then they could have pulled off right where I was standing and run me over. I explained my situation.

"I think you belong about seven miles back at the Number 6 Truck Stop," one of them told me. "We'll help hide your bicycle in the bushes and take you back there."

An anxious Edna welcomed her wandering vagabond. The officers, John Santistevan and Russ Bullington, turned around and headed east again. Edna and I were quickly back on the road to search for my hidden bicycle. In the darkness it was hard to tell exactly where we were. Then, just as we reached the right place, there stood our two good Samaritan state troopers with their powerful spotlight focused on the bicycle. Sometimes I would go for days without seeing these "keepers of the peace," but tonight, when I had lost my way, they had stopped within feet of where I stood!

The next day Edna took me back to milepost 74 to chalk off more miles. Then she went on into Deming to fill the water and gas tanks, buy supplies, and stop at the post office. While there, she also talked to the newspaper office, then caught up with me in Akela Flats. I came aboard to rest a few minutes just before 11:00 a.m. I had 36 miles behind me and wanted to get back on the road until noon.

At lunch time I smelled the aroma before I reached the van. Edna had fixed baked potatoes, peas, vegetarian steaks (made from soya or wheat products), salad, and bread. I have been a vegetarian for 50 years, take no supplements or medicine, have high bone density, and have never had major surgery. With enough energy for two people, I knew this was the lifestyle for me. It felt wonderful to be alive!

Late in the day we stopped at a campground near Las Cruces. How wonderful to have a hot shower, wash my now less-than-white hair, and make a phone call or two. I had gone 69.5 miles that day, passing through barren desert, irrigated farm lands, and open plains.

A dark cloud began to form on our happy horizon. Edna called her husband, Demil, who wanted her to come home the following week. I had hoped to have her with me longer, but knew that whatever happened was for the best. I decided to call Janine, who had originally planned to travel with me before she became ill. Maybe she could come and drive. I dialed Janine's number—but *my husband* answered.

"I have been praying for two days that you would call," he said. "I sent all your mail to the post office in Fabens, Texas. I was so afraid that you would miss the pick-up."

We would be going through Fabens, just 30 miles from El Paso, the next day. If the telephone wires hadn't "gotten crossed," we would not have known to stop for the mail! That night we parked beside a church and were soon sound asleep.

TO YOUR HEALTH!

Before we start across Texas, let's talk about the "E" in FRESH START, which stands for Exercise. *Exercise increases the general circulation, decreases the risk of heart attack by one-half, and decreases the pulse rate, giving the heart more time to rest, while bringing more oxygen to the body. Someone once stated, "Activity is the law of life; idleness the law of death." Exercise makes you feel better, think clearly, relax, develop a better self-image, sleep better, and builds stronger bones. Why, then, do millions never exercise at all?*

Walking is the best all-around exercise, especially when done outdoors in the morning air and sunshine. It aids digestion, strengthens the liver, kidneys, and lungs, and improves the circulation.

Put exercise in your schedule early in the day, if possible, as the metabolic rate stays higher, thus burning more calories. Let's turn stagnation into action!

At 8:00 the next morning the sky was clear. Less than two hours later the wind had whipped up, and I found myself in the middle of one of those dreaded sandstorms. Forty-mile-an-hour side winds kept knocking me off my bike. Blowing sand pelted my eyes and peppered my arms and legs. I had never been in weather like that! Edna stayed close behind me, and when the bike refused to go anymore, I put it on the rack. Afraid that the van might blow over, I told Edna to find shelter. Bending forward to protect my face, I continued to walk. The next day the paper reported wind gusts of up to 54 miles per hour. That wind had blown the roof off a building and the windshield out of a car.

I made only 23 miles that day, but I had walked into Texas. We parked at the Texas information center for the night. In the morning we would embark on an adventure across the biggest state in the Union.

ACROSS TEXAS

I had been on the road nearly three weeks. As we followed the Rio Grande River toward El Paso, we passed through vast pecan groves. Although nuts are higher in fat than grains, fruit, and vegetables, they have a very important place in the diet. Recent studies at Loma Linda University show that people who eat a few nuts a day, five times a week, have less heart disease and are thinner.

Near El Paso the sky became unbelievably bright. Dark clouds gathered, their edges shining like gold from the sun behind them. Silence covered the landscape. I focused my eyes on the heavens as I rode. Suddenly I heard it—not an audible voice, but still a clear statement: "I will take care of you." Only God knew the experiences ahead that would test my faith. Only He knew that bandits would chase me in Nepal, or that I would enter forbidden territory in China. From that moment I received great comfort, knowing I would have a Guide to show me the way and protect me from danger.

Edna picked up our mail at Fabens. How great to get a little news from home! As we continued through farm and ranch lands I rode for miles, seeing few signs of life. I covered 71 miles for the day.

From Fort Hancock I started for Van Horn. I had become adept at dodging around equipment and roadblocks and handling the bumpy road during the many miles of road construction I encountered. Sometimes I allowed myself the luxury of riding on a newly paved area that was not yet open to traffic. Unfortunately, Edna's impending departure overshadowed the joy of the day, so after 64 miles we checked in at a KOA camp, thankful for hot showers and an electrical hook-up.

Edna was to fly out of Abilene, a day's travel away. Taking her to the airport and returning would mean the loss of two days of riding for me. When I mentioned my concern to the camp's desk clerk, he said, "Why, there's a bus leaving from downtown, just a few blocks from here, at 7:00 in the morning." Edna could ride the bus to the airport!

We spent our last evening talking about the good times we'd enjoyed together. After the bus left the next morning I came back to the park alone. I missed my friend already. And I still faced the problem of finding a driver for the Mini-Cruiser. Dorothy and Gene were both searching for someone, but so far without success. I knew I must put my faith in God. He knew the whole picture.

Dreary, miserable weather dominated the day, including a strong, northeast wind. I decided to clean the camper and ended up packing two boxes of items to send home. Next, I tackled the laundry. The activity and sense of order helped to lift my spirits. A family from Germany, whom I had met earlier, stopped to say goodbye. They had rented an RV and were spending part of their vacation traveling from Oceanside (where I had started) to Corpus Christi. The father and his two sons rode racing bicycles, while the mother and daughter drove the RV. What a handsome, physically fit family!

All was ready for the next day, except I hadn't figured out how to drive my van and ride a bicycle at the same time! The situation seemed impossible. That evening I stopped at the Texaco station in town and asked the manager, Chevel Alvarado, if I could park overnight and leave my vehicle there the next day. I planned to ride ahead on my bicycle, then return in the evening to pick up the van.

"I'll do one better," he smiled. "My wife and I are going shopping at Pecos tomorrow. We'll pick you up at Kent on our way home."

I thanked him, then parked the van in back of the station. I thanked God for His continuing care over me before quickly falling fast asleep between my freshly-laundered sheets.

I was on the road the next morning by 7:20, running ahead of a strong tailwind. I reached Kent by 10:20, covering 37 miles along a route that included lots of climbing! My leg muscles, growing stronger every day, had proved equal to the task. A conversation with Mike Tyrrell, manager of a combination garage-grocery store, resulted in an invitation to leave my bicycle there while I went back for the camper. About an hour later, Chevel and his wife picked me up for the ride back to Van Horn. He pointed out homesteads and landmarks along the way that had looked like only open range and lifeless scenery to me as I rode through it earlier in the day.

When I returned to Mike's garage, he greeted me with good news. His mother-in-law, Pauline, would take my van ahead to Toyah, 32 miles east of Kent, my weekend stop. His wife, Tammy, would pick up her mother to bring her back home. Although it was Pauline's first experience of driving an RV, I felt no concern. This whole experience was a faith venture! We met at a truck stop in Toyah. I will never forget their kindness and help. I traveled 69 miles that Friday!

I spent a quiet weekend parked beside a Texaco station in Toyah. Sunday morning the temperature dropped to 20 degrees, and a driving snow was falling outside my camper. I decided to wait and hope for better weather on Monday.

Travis Heald, the station's owner, came by during the afternoon. The big man removed his 10-gallon hat, revealing a shock of white hair. His life had taken a tragic turn six years earlier, when a warning shot he fired into the air accidentally hit and partially paralyzed a thief who had left without paying for his gas. After six years of probation for the shooting, Travis now faced a $1 million lawsuit filed by the thief.

"So much has gone wrong because of this," he said. "Even my wife left me."

When I traveled through the area some time later, the new manager said Travis had passed away after a heart attack. I wonder what happened to the thief? I hope he found a better way of life.

Monday morning I dressed in several layers, then added my down coat for good measure. As I was checking the tires on the bike, two women and a big man got out of two large trucks parked nearby. Just as they passed me I said under my breath, "How I wish there was someone to drive my support van east so that I could ride my bike."

The trio kept right on walking into the Texaco station. I finished with the tires and went inside.

"Do you really mean what you said outside?" one of the women asked.

"I surely do," came my quick and firm reply.

"How do you know that I won't just keep going on down the road?"

"Do you believe in prayer?" I questioned.

"I surely do!"

We introduced ourselves. All three, Dee, Betty, and the gentleman, were Bell Telephone employees, driving unmarked trucks to pick up money from phone meters. Betty, a new employee, had accompanied Dee to learn the ropes.

When we left, Betty was driving Dee's truck and Dee was driving in my van, headed east to Penwell. I would call her when I arrived. Inside my van was a public-address system, a slide projector, camera, tape recorder, and other equipment. Yet I felt perfectly safe in turning the whole thing over to her. I learned later that Dee was licensed to drive any vehicle on the road, including 18-wheelers.

I had forgotten my water bottle that morning, so about midday I stopped at the West Texas Children's Home for water and a meal break. When the principal asked me to speak to the youngsters, I welcomed the opportunity.

"Don't think about the things you can't help," I told them. "Focus on what you can do. Set a goal for yourselves and go for it. I lost my van driver when another nurse, who was going to walk and ride with me, got pneumonia. Instead of giving up I went right ahead planning my trip. Now here I am with this 15-speed touring Schwinn Marada and a good-looking, blue-and-white helmet with a visor to keep the sun off. Most of my gear were gifts, things I couldn't afford to buy. God knows I'm out here, and He cares about me, just like He cares about you. Follow the rules so that you can go back home and help your parents and be useful happy young men. You can do anything you want to do if you don't give up."

Perhaps it was providential that I had forgotten my water bottle. It gave me the opportunity to share with a group of young men who were searching for a direction in life. By the end of the day I had ridden 88 miles, in addition to talking to the boys.

Not only did Trucker Dee drive my van, she insisted that I sleep in her home. That night I drove the van and followed Dee and her husband, John, in their car to their home in Odessa. After a delicious supper of salad and steamed vegetables, I enjoyed a wonderful soak in a tub of hot water before I went to bed. I awoke the next morning to find my clothes on the dresser, washed and folded. Dee's husband fed me breakfast, then took me back to Penwell.

Leaving the van in Penwell, I once more peddled eastward. I had gone about five miles when I realized I couldn't remember if I had closed the side door of the van. Going back to check meant 10 miles of riding. What should I do? I decided not to go back and prayed for the safety of my new typewriter and other valuables as I continued to ride.

I felt a need to call Gene around 2:00 that afternoon. When he answered, excitement filled his voice. "Dorothy says Blanche Meidel will come drive for you, but if you'd like her to join you, her ticket must be paid for today."

Would I! Dorothy volunteered to pay for Blanche's ticket, and I made plans to pick her up in Abilene. Blanche had been part of a group I recruited in 1967 for a tour of the Holy Land. We had joined a larger group sponsored by the well-known radio program *Voice of Prophecy*. I looked forward to having her with me.

Betty (Trucker Dee's partner) had invited me to have supper with her and her husband, Bill Barnhill, that evening at their country place in Stanton. After supper Bill went out to look at my bike. "Charlotte," he called, "you have a flat tire!"

The cause of the trouble? A big Texas thorn! I was so glad it hadn't happened out on a country road as darkness approached. Bill patched the tire and put some sealant inside the tube.

I hadn't mentioned my concern about the door on the camper, but the Barnhills decided it would be wise to take me back to the van that evening, since Bill worked at the Confederate Air Force Base and had to leave at 2:30 a.m. When we pulled up, the side door of the camper was swinging freely in the breeze! What if I hadn't returned until the next day and the door had remained open during the night? How very much I appreciated these caring Texans. Bill and Betty had driven nearly 108 miles, round-trip, to bring me back to Penwell. My prayers of gratitude flew heavenward many times a day, but that night I was especially thankful. I hadn't needed to use my emergency tire kit out on the road, Blanche was coming, and I was safe inside an intact vehicle.

I drove the Mini-Cruiser to Stanton the next morning, April Fool's Day, and parked it at a FINA station. Then I started another day of traveling alone on the road, cycling from Stanton toward Colorado City. The countryside changed as I covered the miles. I rode by many shut-down oil wells. The working wells looked like great birds, endlessly moving their beaks up and down, pulling the oil from the bowels of the earth. Rusting oil well parts lay in great stockpiles. A sea of dry grass surrounded the silent towns where the doors of empty buildings with crumbling plaster walls swung on squeaky hinges.

I enjoyed listening to tapes as I rode. A commentary of about 20 tapes on Daniel and Revelation, plus the entire Bible, helped to pass the time. Most of all, though, they strengthened and prepared me for things yet to come. The commentary's author, Dr. Graham Maxwell, had been a teacher in the Religion Department at Loma Linda University. (His father, Arthur Maxwell, wrote the well-known children's books *Uncle Arthur's Bedtime Stories* and *The Bible Story.*)

The grass beside the roadside began to look greener. More ponds dotted the countryside, and herds of Angus cattle grazed peacefully in the fields. I stopped at Bill's Truck Stop in Colorado City. I needed to find a way back to Stanton to get the van. Bill, the owner, offered me a ride, but I would have to wait until he finished at the station later in the day.

I decided to go to a nearby restaurant. Troy Smith, the host, invited me to enjoy a meal as their guest. He also called the local radio station. Reporter Jim Baum came over and interviewed me while I ate. Sometimes people could not believe what I was doing, riding alone on those wild plains and forsaken deserts. "And for what?" was the unspoken question written on their faces.

I made arrangements to leave my bike at the truck stop until the next day. Then the phone rang. It was Troy. A local teacher, Debbie Goforth, who had passed me as I left the restaurant, was offering to take me back to Stanton if I would agree to talk to her students the next morning. (She confessed later she also asked a nurse friend to come with us, in case I might kidnap her or do some bodily harm!) What a pleasure to visit with the two of them after those long hours alone on the road. The trip back to Stanton took more than an hour. Sometimes even I couldn't understand how I had covered all those miles!

At the park that night I moved the van beside another trailer so I wouldn't feel that I was the only frog in the pond. I'm sure it didn't make any difference to God whether I was alone or with other human beings. Either way, I had to trust Him to take care of me. At 11:30 a violent wind blast suddenly hit the camper, shaking the small vehicle back and forth, much like a cat shakes a mouse. Sand, whipped by the wind, peppered the sides. For a moment fear enveloped me. Was it a tornado? I don't remember ever experiencing such a sudden manifestation of nature's power—power I was helpless to resist.

Up by 6:15 the next morning, I phoned Blanche to tell her what to bring—rather, what *not* to bring. "Leave nearly everything at home. There are enough linens and everything we need here for both of us. I don't know how to tell you, but be assured you are the answer to all my prayers. See you Friday!"

I drove the Mini-Cruiser to Debbie's school in Colorado City. Her classroom was jammed to the doors. Other classes and teachers had also come to hear me speak. I had my bike with me, plus all the gear that goes with it—gloves, helmet, shoes, whistle, lock keys around my neck, and earphones for the cassette player on my belt. My white hair contrasted sharply with the tan I had acquired from days in the sun. My figure has changed little since age 17, and I still move just about as fast. I was definitely not what they expected to see in a grandmother.

"I'm on the road to encourage people to make good choices so that they won't get sick and have headaches and feel tired and discouraged so much of the time," I told my young audience. "I ride this bike from 50 to 80 miles a day and still have enough energy to go for a walk in the evening. My bones are strong, I don't take any medicine, and I haven't had any major surgery. I feel good and I'm happy, because I hope to live and do what I want to do until I'm 100 years old!"

A real human heart, a lung, and some clogged arteries I had brought with me fascinated the students. I held up long, spaghetti-like pieces of fat. "Most of you have some streaks of fat on the walls of your blood vessels already. If you live on burgers, French fries, and milkshakes, which are loaded with cholesterol and fat, you could eventually have one or more arteries entirely closed. No blood would be able to get through to carry food and oxygen and take away the waste from the cells. Learn to enjoy fruits, vegetables, and whole-grain cereals. They have no cholesterol and very little fat. Get out and walk or play. Do something useful every day. You can feel good, have clean arteries, and always have lots of energy. It's up to you."

I showed them the lung. "Look at this black lung. It should be about the color of your face. See this large white area? That's a tumor. Smoking killed the man who owned this lung. Don't start smoking or drinking.

"Do you have something that you would really like to do? If it is not selfish and will help others, go for it! Dream and work toward it every day, and your dream will come true."

The whole school came outside to say goodbye. Debbie told me they had made a tape of my presentation. Students would be able to hear my message long after I had gone on down the road.

A strong wind gusted from the northeast as I started out on the interstate. Forty-five minutes later I had gone only one mile. Enough is enough, I decided, and returned to MacMichael's Restaurant, where I had stopped the day before. Sitting at a table to one side, I used the time to catch up my journal. I had food in the camper, but the delicious smells from the kitchen were overpowering. After a baked potato, salad, and a piece of coconut pie I was full! (A piece of pie now and then adds a little zest to living, don't you think?)

About 6:00 p.m. I pulled into the Oasis Campground a few miles from Abilene. Blanche would arrive at the Abilene airport the next morning. I vacuumed and did some cleaning. After a shower and a prayer of thanks for all the blessings of the past week, I fell fast asleep.

NOT ALONE ANYMORE

When I arrived at the Abilene airport, I discovered that Blanche's flight was late. So I rushed back to the campground for a press interview with a KTAB TV reporter, who stayed nearly an hour, filming me as I rode. Then Don Blakley from the Abilene *Reporter* stayed nearly another hour. By now the news media were getting to know about me, and I considered them part of my team.

Back at the airport again I felt a little anxious. Blanche and I had not seen each other for 20 years. Would we recognize each other? Then I saw her, smiling, blue eyes flashing confidence in a new challenge, and all those years evaporated in a big bear hug!

By midafternoon I took to the wheels again, beginning where the wind had stopped me the day before. I advanced 27 miles and felt thankful it was Friday. I looked forward to 24 hours away from the noise and exhaust fumes from thousands of semis and cars, not to mention the glass, nails, and ripped-up tires that sometimes littered the road. We stopped at Rolling Hills Campground in Sweetwater, Texas. When the campground owners invited us to stay for the weekend as their guests, we knew another blessing had fallen upon us.

A strong wind still blew from the east Sunday morning, so we spent the day in the campground. Between phone calls, reports home, and log entries, we had lots to do, including falling asleep in the middle of the morning. When we walked to the nearby truck stop in the evening, two truckers offered to install a citizen's band radio in the van for us. This army of men and women who passed me in their 18-wheelers had become a familiar part of my journey. As they thundered down the interstate in rigs that seemed to reach to the heavens, I would be literally stopped in my tracks when they passed me. Sometimes they carried me along with the wind they generated. Some of them thought I was crazy to be out there. Others remarked, "She has lots of guts!" Not very flowery language, but I called them my guardian angels of the road, and they tracked me on their CB radios. I knew that their help was there if I needed it.

They often tooted to encourage me as they went by. I waved in reply and thanked them in the media for giving me space. While semis usually moved over to another lane for me, buses and RVs sometimes came dangerously close. Cattle trucks never budged; they had to stay fairly steady to keep from throwing the cattle from side to side. Same for tankers. A sudden turn of the wheel would set the liquid in tankers in motion. So I had to keep alert and be ready for anything. Sometimes I dared not even listen to my tapes.

We left the campground early Monday morning with good weather and a tolerable wind. I biked up and down rolling hills all day, arriving back at the Oasis Campground by early afternoon. KORQ radio and KTXA television reporters met us there. An hour passed before I was back on the road.

We rolled into the quaint town of Putnam at 7:00 p.m. Townspeople welcomed us into their circle as if we belonged there, and a pleasant gentleman invited us to park by his pecan grove for the night. I especially remember Ida Mae Waddington, a delightful older resident and Putnam's justice of the peace, who invited us to visit her home. The old clock in the parlor seemed to tick off the lateness of the hour for folks who had once been young and full of hope and adventure.

It was late when we arrived back at the pecan grove. My legs had pushed out 78 miles that day, and we had taken time with the press. Out under the stars the soft night sounds played through the pecan trees as we drifted off to dreamland.

After breakfast the next morning I couldn't resist one backward glance at the little town. It may have lost its hold on progress with its unpaved roads and weather-beaten buildings. What it did have, though, was lots of friendly people.

We had lunch in Eastland. The young woman behind the counter of the Smoke Stack Cafe told us that 60,000 people had once lived there. Now only 60 remained. All along the way the little towns seemed deserted and forgotten.

The landscape turned greener and more flowers dotted the countryside. This was, however, still Texas—yesterday, today, and tomorrow. I told Blanche, "If I ever get out of Texas it shouldn't be much farther to the Atlantic!" And those *long, long* hills—not steep, but steadily up-grade, then *swish!* a few seconds going down, with not even time to catch a breath before I started climbing again.

The next day we traveled from Santo to Fort Worth. Before we left I called Mark at WXTZ in Charleston, South Carolina, to tell him I was still on the road and heading his way. He was keeping his radio audience posted on my progress.

Out on the freeway a patrolman stopped me for riding in the right lane. I rode there because of the rough shoulder, but promised him I'd obey his instructions to stay on the shoulder. Thankfully, the condition of the shoulder soon improved.

At noon Blanche had lunch ready in Weatherford, where she had also picked up the mail. But we missed each other somehow. While Blanche waited, I sped down the interstate toward Fort Worth, a city of gleaming skyscrapers and nearly a half million people. Somehow I ended up on the main artery going into the city.

"Keep me safe up here, Lord," I prayed. "Don't let these speeding semis crowd me too close. And if there isn't room for them and me on the bridge at the same time, hold them back until I get on the other side."

Where should I get off the expressway? I turned right and headed down below the main highway onto the service road. I spotted a Schwinn bike shop and pulled in. While the young man adjusted the brakes and inspected the bike, I bought a burrito, some honey pudding, and pillow bread at a nearby Mexican restaurant. Just as I stepped back onto the service road, I spotted Blanche in the heavy traffic above, inching her way forward. I did a 50-yard dash and caught her. I can't call it anything but another answered prayer.

That night we stayed in a room at the Seventh-day Adventist college in Keene, Texas. I enjoyed visiting with Eleanor, a former faculty member from Andrews University Nursing Department, and some of my former students. After the heat, smog, and clouds of dust, it felt wonderful to be clean again and in fresh clothes. Blanche and I slept soundly, reunited once more, safe and sound.

By 10:00 the next morning we were back in Fort Worth. We made 50 copies of newspaper articles and materials to use along the way as press kits. We spent part of the afternoon at Huguley Hospital. Shirley Pinterick and one of my former nursing students, who had attended one of my workshops at Andrews, were holding workshops and screenings for a Prevent the 3 Cs course I had developed for student nurses. Clients from several counties came to hear the students lecture and learn how to reduce risks that predispose to coronary, cancer, and C.V.A. (stroke). Shirley asked me to speak to the 30 nurses on duty who filled the little chapel. They seemed very interested in what I was doing, some saying they wished they could do it, too. I think most people dream of traveling to some faraway place, or of accomplishing something unusual. All too often it never happens.

That afternoon reporters from the Crowley *Eagle* and the Burleson *Star* interviewed me. The article and accompanying picture in the next day's *Star* took up nearly half the front page. The caption stated "Charlotte Hamlin, 68-year-old retired nurse, stopped at Huguley Memorial Hospital last Thursday on her way across the country, to give a talk. She hopes to demonstrate that anyone at any age can be healthy." It would take many lectures to reach as many people as read the story in just one newspaper or heard it on a television or radio broadcast.

And the day wasn't over yet! Several classrooms of children and their teachers waited for me under an overpass. I almost tipped over as my bike skidded to a stop in the loose shale by the roadside.

"Learn all you can now while you have the chance," I told them. "You usually know what the right choice is when a decision has to be made. What you decide now and every day determines what is going to happen to you 20 years from now. Why not build your body with strong and healthy materials so it won't fall apart in a few years? I wouldn't be here talking to you if I just ate French fries and potato chips and milk shakes and soft drinks. They don't make good blood, and they are not good fuel for pedaling a bicycle."

After teaching for years I know that it's not so much what you tell others to do as what they see you doing that makes the lasting impression.

"Do you stay up late and watch TV? Your body has to make protein and other important things while you sleep. You may not grow to your full height if you stay up late. You won't feel as good inside the next day, either. Each one of you is important, so be sure to take care of yourself. Thanks for coming out here on the road. Meeting you makes the time pass quicker and makes the Atlantic Ocean seem a little closer."

The youngsters looked so young and healthy as they sat there. I hoped they would make wise decisions about their health as they grew older.

It was Friday again. Back on the road by 9:00 a.m. in hot weather and heavy traffic, I found leaving Fort Worth on Highway 35W quite challenging. Riding a bicycle down a road without any handicaps is sometimes unpredictable. In the middle of noise and hurry, squeezed for space, the going is unbelievably hazardous. As I approached a bridge with a very narrow shoulder, I heard an almost audible command: "Don't go on the bridge!"

Just as I turned my head, a semi shot past me and onto the bridge. When I rode onto the bridge after that bolt of steel blazed by, I could see that my handlebars were wider than the shoulder! Had I gone on the bridge a moment sooner . . . Well, I hate to think about it.

Blanche had dinner ready at noon. During the day she checked public relations, bought food for the weekend, cleaned, and took care of other needs. What a woman! In her 50s, Blanche has short hair and is short of stature, but such a big heart! She took pictures, went anywhere, and did anything to keep the wheels turning toward the eastern border of Texas.

Dallas is another big city—about twice as big as Fort Worth. The city bulged with activity. By 5:30 p.m. my bicycle wheels stopped turning at milepost 492. I would start here again on Sunday morning. With the bicycle on the rack, we rode in the van to Terrel and stayed at Terry's 24-Hour STOP. Even though 70 miles of riding lay behind me for the day, Blanche and I took a short walk that evening.

The next day we joined 20 or 30 other people for worship in a little church. When invited to speak, I talked about how good health coordinates with the good life. If we have pain in our body, become depressed in our mind, or feel unrest in our spirit, it doesn't matter how rich we are, how many friends we have, or how intelligent we happen to be, we would do anything to feel better.

A lovely, middle-aged couple invited us to visit their country home, located about nine miles from the church. We also visited the farm owned by the church's song leader, an 85-year-old gentleman. A lonely widower, he had also lost his daughter and lived alone on the farm. About 8:00 that evening we returned to the church, where I enjoyed playing old hymns and choruses on the organ. It was a good soother of body, mind, and spirit at the end of another week on the road.

Sunday morning we returned to Forney, about seven miles back toward Dallas, to begin where I had stopped on Friday. Despite the sunshine, the wind made me aware that I wasn't always entirely in charge of how many miles I would travel in a day. As I turned off the freeway at Colfax, about 48 miles down the road, a tall, handsome gentleman with dark hair and clean-cut features waited at the entrance of the rest area.

"Could I talk to you?" he asked.

John Freeman (not his real name) had done some cycling in the past. The ACROSS AMERICA sign around my waist intrigued him. In his early 40s, he had two seminary degrees from different universities and a Ph.D. in psychology. Obviously concerned about something, he reminded me of Nicodemus who came to Christ at night to find out what he needed to do to find peace in his life.

Two years earlier John had held his wife in his arms as she died from cancer. The sad parts of life continually passed before him in his work as a psychologist. Loneliness threatened to overwhelm him. He had taken a Daniel and Revelation seminar from a Seventh-day Adventist church and considered it a highlight in his life, saying he now had a better focus in his life. But there still remained a vacuum somewhere. If only there were some way to fill a basket with faith, the kind that gives us confidence that God knows all about it and will see us through. Then we could break off pieces and pass it around to those in need. We visited for about an hour, then promised to meet him two days later as we traveled east. He wanted to arrange some television and newspaper interviews.

An angry sky and a tornado warning greeted us the next morning. The wind howled, thunder rolled, and flashes of lightning filled the sky as the storm poured heavy rain down upon us. We stayed inside until the storm passed. Before long, sunshine beckoned me back to the road.

As we pulled into a rest stop near the Longview-Marshall area, something about the place made me uneasy. Blanche and I walked across the road to use the telephone at a rest area for traffic going the other direction. A Mrs. Smith greeted us, concerned about our safety.

"Come over here and park in this area. It's not open to the public, but we're living here in a trailer," she told us. "My husband is in charge of repair work going on here."

Mr. Smith looked a young 60, the result of no worries and hard work outdoors. He hooked up our camper with one of his extension cords and emptied both holding tanks. He filled our clean water tank before we left the next day. With the battery recharged and everything serviced, I felt recharged too and pedaled 71 miles before taking off my helmet for the day.

We weren't far from Kilgore, the center of the vast East Texas oil fields, where oil had been discovered in 1930. At one time more than 1,100 oil wells had operated within the city limits, 24 of them in the downtown area on an acre of land known as the world's richest acre. That spot is a park today.

Cool weather greeted us the next morning, and a northwest wind blew all day. Because of road construction, only one lane of the highway was open most of the time. We had lunch in Texas; then, believe it or not, we left the Lone Star State at last! At 1:00 we crossed the border into Louisiana and stopped at a visitors' center that bubbled with congeniality. The *Times,* a Gannett newspaper in Shreveport, came out for an interview and pictures.

We were getting closer and closer to the finish line. I called Thousand Oaks, California, to find out when the *Christian Lifestyle* television crew, who planned to film a documentary about my trip, would meet us. We agreed to join them on April 30 in Atlanta.

Interstate 20 took me through Shreveport, a city of more than 200,000 people. As usual, bridges presented the most danger be-

TO YOUR HEALTH!

Before we travel farther we need to explore another letter in our FRESH START *acronym. We've made it as far as "S," which stands for* Simple diet.

In our country millions struggle to lose weight. They fight the fear of breast cancer, take something for headaches, or check their blood sugar because of diabetes. The easiest way to get back on track is to get out and exercise, eat the food God gave our first parents (fruits, grains, nuts, and vegetables), and ask Him to help us take advantage of a more natural diet. A little milk and an occasional egg probably won't upset the apple cart; however, we know that animal products contain large amounts of cholesterol and triglycerides. To complicate matters, we add sugar, fat, salt, spices, chemicals, and color to our diet with cookies, cakes, ice cream, and more. There are foods, simply prepared, that taste just as delicious and that give more energy, as well as protecting the immune system.

I'm not saying we all have to be vegetarians, but wisdom dictates that we would enjoy life more if we leaned in that direction. Most of all, though, don't become discouraged and quit. Just choose the best way one day at a time.

cause of the narrow shoulders. I had to spill right out into the main traffic lane. I must have had an angel at both elbows. Attacking these big cities instead of going around them shortened the time, though, and I suppose everybody needs a challenge now and then. Watching the signs, figuring out which lane to get into (and when to simply get out of the way) kept the excitement high. Back on the open road once more I relaxed and enjoyed the panoramic view of green fields, feeding egrets, and well-groomed horses grazing in the pastures.

A swollen and painful left knee troubled me as I walked around that evening. When I phoned my older brother that evening, I mentioned the knee. As president of industrial medicine for Western Canada he had the answer. "Keep your foot straight ahead on the pedal," he advised. "You're lifting your knee up and down with your foot out of alignment." So I positioned my foot straight on the pedal the next day and the problem was solved almost immediately.

While I rode along the freeway, Blanche drove to Minden to mail some cards. We met for a dinner of mung beans, Chinese beans we had soaked several days, let sprout, and then put in salads or ate as they were. They taste a little like raw green peas and are very nourishing, containing a good amount of minerals, Vitamin C, and other vitamins. We added steam-fried potatoes and onions, salad, and yellow squash. As we enjoyed our meal, I told Blanche about the patrolman who had stopped me that morning on the freeway.

"It's all right for you to stay on," he had said. "I'm not going to be the one to make you get off!"

I rode all afternoon, and that evening after supper I talked myself into riding some more. A new freeway, not yet open to the public, looked like smooth, black velvet as I glided over it through the evening hours. When we stopped at a campground in Monroe, my cycle and I had rolled out 70 miles for the day.

The next day proved to be one of the biggest media days so far. We enjoyed a visit with John Freeman, who had also brought a friend who was interested in what we were doing. (Maybe John *had* gotten a little piece of faith out of the basket!) John had notified the press, and a steady stream of interviewers visited us. Zero miles on the road, but a busy, productive day nevertheless.

CROSSING THE MISSISSIPPI

Between Monroe and Vicksburg lay some of the flattest terrain of the entire trip. And if I hadn't ridden over so many mountains I wouldn't have appreciated it half so much! Maybe that's what hardships accomplish—they help us to be more thankful for the easier times. I left the freeway just moments before Blanche arrived at our meeting point with a pizza for lunch. I'm not too enthusiastic about cheese, especially the high-fat, aged kind. Pizza can, however, taste good and add variety if you use low-fat Mozzarella or ricotta (farmer's) cheese. Vegetables used in place of some of the cheese reduce calories and add flavor.

We ate beside a shimmering lake, home to a group of mallard ducks. As we rested I reflected on how nature brings peace and contentment into our lives. That afternoon we visited the Delhi post office. The post mistress seemed delighted that we had stopped by. A lady walked in and gave us a copy of the Monroe paper that had a big story about our journey and mission.

I had 68 miles behind me for the day when I joined Blanche in the van that evening. We crossed over the Mississippi River and stopped in a little park in Vicksburg. Tomorrow we would rest. With the mighty Mississippi River at our feet and the sun slowly disappearing below the horizon, we bowed our heads in gratitude and praise for the One who created us and this beautiful world.

At church the next day, who should I see but John Evans, M.D., an old acquaintance. We had met when John visited Andrews University Nursing Department. He's the one who lent me the human heart that I displayed with my talks.

Sunday morning I resumed my trip at mile marker 185 at the Louisiana Travel Bureau. I knew that the long Mississippi River bridge waited ahead of me. "Calm down, Charlotte," I said under my breath. "You have made it over more than bridges. What makes you think this obstacle will be any different?"

A group of school children dressed in red shirts and khaki pants had come to meet me with their bikes. They wanted to accompany me for a ways out on the freeway, but I was afraid someone might get hurt. We did take some pictures, though. A teacher and an X-ray technician who had accompanied the children rode with me across the bridge. Even though traffic was almost nil, I rode as if a bear were chasing me and reached the other side before I knew it. Often the things we worry about are not half so serious as they seem. Only about eight percent of the things we worry about need to be worked through, and most of the rest either don't happen or work themselves out without our help.

I was on the freeway once more, through Vicksburg, and ready to see what other worlds I would need to conquer. Claude Atkins, a park ranger, had told us he was very hesitant to let me ride on the freeway. A recent serious accident during a benefit walk-a-thon had left six people dead. For some reason he allowed me to proceed anyway.

Construction work at Pearl River slowed our progress. At dusk we pulled into Bob's Magnolia RV Park, having clocked 50 miles

TO YOUR HEALTH!

As we cross the Mississippi we must say something about **Happiness**, *the "H" in* **FRESH START**. *The Bible tells us much about happiness. "A heart at peace gives life to the body, but envy rots the bones" (Prov. 14:30, NIV). "Pleasant words are a honeycomb, sweet to the soul and healing to the bones" (Prov. 16:24, NIV). "A cheerful heart is good medicine, but a crushed spirit dries up the bones" (Prov. 17:22, NIV).*

Red blood cells are made in the long bones. The life is in the blood, and a happy disposition helps to keep the blood healthy, too.

Being happy is important. In her book Ministry of Healing, *Ellen White states, "The relation that exists between the mind and the body is very intimate. When one is affected, the other sympathizes. The condition of the mind affects the health to a far greater degree than many realize. Many of the diseases from which men suffer are the result of mental depression. Grief, anxiety, discontent, remorse, guilt, distrust, all tend to break down the life forces and to invite decay and death. . . . Courage, hope, faith, sympathy, love, promote health and prolong life" (p. 241). How wonderful that each of us can choose the route we wish to take!*

for the day. We didn't have a TV to watch the interview we'd done earlier, but a neighboring camper graciously agreed to let us watch on his set.

On Monday, April 20, we took our camper in for a service check. Everything was in good condition, and by 11:00 a.m. I was on the road again. I saw a pickup stopped on the shoulder of the road ahead of me. A young man came to the back of the vehicle and signaled for me to stop. He held a copy of the newspaper article about my trip in his hand and told me how happy he felt at finding me on the road. He seemed very distraught, however, so I asked him if something was troubling him.

He almost cried as he answered. "My wife doesn't want to be married anymore. She says it's not my fault—she just wants to be alone. I love her very much. What can I do?"

We talked for some time. "She knows you love her," I said finally, "so just do your best to fill your place as a partner and ask God to take over where you cannot." Then we prayed together out there on the road. I still pray for him and often wonder what happened.

We parked along the freeway at lunchtime. As we were eating, two women drove up and came to the door of the van. "We have gone east on this freeway for miles," one of them said excitedly. "And then we went west for a good spell, then back this way twice, looking for you. When we saw your picture and the write-up in the newspaper, we just had to find you."

Susan Carrell and Sharon Bordon, two businesswomen out for a little adventure, talked with us about our mission and how worthwhile our trip had been thus far. They gave us some nice little gifts before they left.

It was almost 3:00 before the rubber met the road again, and both the rubber and the road were sizzling hot! Waves of heat shimmered up from the pavement. Pouring water down my neck and over my body cooled me temporarily. Catching a little breeze coming toward me as I rode also acted as a temporary cooler, especially if my clothes were wet. A little sympathy seemed in order, even it if came from myself! Fortunately, this kind of day didn't happen too frequently. Even in the heat, however, it felt good to chalk off the miles.

Early the next morning I phoned Gene to give a progress update, then back out into the sun and the sharp rocks on the shoulder of the road again. It's a wonder the rocks didn't tear the bike's tires to shreds, but they rode over the rocks very well—better than I did, I might add. Finally, I was back on the edge of the freeway. We stopped early for dinner and parked on the side of the road near Hickory. A highway trooper came to the door with a message.

"A Pastor Jack Nash and some school children are looking for you," he said. He never said a word about our being on the freeway.

We eventually met up with Pastor Nash and his group and enjoyed a nice visit. The children stared at me in disbelief. I wasn't exactly the kind of grandmother they had expected to meet.

By 12:30 I was back on the road where the temperature reached 95 degrees and broke all records for April. I don't suppose the humidity was much better. Around 2:00 Channel 11 (WTOK TV in Meridian) caught up with me. Tracy Winchell interviewed me while Ted Davis took pictures. They included Blanche in the story, which I thought was the best so far.

About 6:00 Pauline Dunn, a member of Pastor Nash's group, took us shopping at a local mall. At the athletic store I picked out some tops and shorts, but they wouldn't let me pay for them. After we arrived back at the parked van a lovely young journalist from the Meridian *Star World* interviewed me. In her article she talked about my trust in God, not in myself. The whole piece was very practical and down-to-earth. Later Pauline insisted that we spend the night in her home. After the heat of the road that day it felt super to clean up and wash our clothes. We enjoyed visiting with her in such a homey and relaxing atmosphere and slept soundly that night.

A SCARE IN THE NIGHT

For breakfast Pauline gave us pancakes with applesauce and syrup. She had also mended my handlebar bag. What a girl! By 8:30 Blanche had me back at the Exxon where I had stopped the night before. We planned to meet at the Alabama welcome center.

About 11:00 one of the bicycle's right side cables broke. Realizing I had been using the gears on the right much more than the ones on the left, I made a mental note to change this habit. I called the folks at the Schwinn bicycle shop in Tuscaloosa. They told me to keep riding—they would install a new cable when I arrived.

Alabama welcomed us with lots of heat and a rocky road shoulder. We had crossed one more border and had two more to go. We left the freeway in Livingston to eat dinner. Our meal consisted of "haystacks," made of layers of corn chips, black-eyed peas, tomatoes, lettuce, onions, and a little dressing. Simple food, but nourishing and delicious. Pete and Joy Raymond, missionaries who were back home for a visit, stopped at the camper. They had seen us on TV and were quite excited to find us in person.

In spite of the broken cable, a bumpy road, and a visit along the way, 58 more miles lay behind us when we pulled into North Bend rest stop for the night. A quiet place on the far side of the campground, near the woods and away from the road, provided the perfect parking spot. We thanked God for a gorgeous sunset and the end of another day on the road.

The next morning I phoned Gene before we left. "We're across the border into Alabama," I told him, "doing fine, trying to keep cool, and headed for Tuscaloosa to get a broken cable taken care of." I mentioned the roads in Alabama. "The road construction department really believes in shale for shoulders! For sure, it would certainly wake up a motorist who goes to sleep and veers off the road. The road crew obviously didn't have me in mind when they dumped tons of sharp shale down on the shoulder and imbedded it in cement!" I told him we planned to be in Tuscaloosa by noon. "The hills will be easier to climb with the new cable."

I did arrive in town by noon. At Cycle Path, the Schwinn bicycle shop, skilled hands gave my bike a thorough check, installed a new cable, cleaned the frame, and oiled necessary parts. Once again, I was charged nothing for this service. Despite the heat that left many of the houses and lawns looking a little wilted, everyone was friendly and helpful.

The time came to say goodbye to this place with such a rich past. Given to the Indians in 1809 by the government, it burned

TO YOUR HEALTH!

Let's talk about the second "S" in FRESH START, which stands for Sunshine. Sunshine has a soothing, relaxing effect on the nervous system. It also lowers the heart rate, increases cardiac output, endurance, and strength.

Sunshine reduces lactic acid in the blood, reduces fatigue, and aids digestion. It increases the use of oxygen in the tissues, which is important in stimulating the immune system, especially in the production of antibodies. Many types of cancer cells do not like oxygen. When exposed to a high concentration, they will begin to slow their growth and finally stop altogether. In this indirect way, sunlight may be able to fight against cancer in the tissues.

Of course, when we lie on the beach in the hot sun until we sizzle, the damage can open the door to skin cancer and other problems. But it's rather like selenium: a little, possibly, helps prevent cancer; but too much might cause it. It is much more sensible to expose the skin for a few minutes every day than to turn lobster red on weekends.

A visor on my helmet protects my face when I'm out on the road. Often I have some covering on my arms. When it's hot, though, I do get a lot of exposure to the sun. Sometimes I use a little sunscreen, but in some cases it's possible that the oil adds to the problem.

Light up your life! Arrange curtains and blinds to let sunlight into all rooms daily. Put bedding and clothing out to air regularly. Work, play, and live outdoors as much as possible, protected from overexposure.

four years later following a revolt. Defeat forced the "Black Warriors" to move westward. Settlers from South Carolina came and named the community Tuscaloosa. It continued to prosper, and the University of Alabama was established in 1831. Many of the town's antebellum houses still stand today.

That night we drove back to the North Bend rest stop. The 30-plus miles for the day weren't anything to write home about, but what we accomplished was perhaps more important than just distance covered. At bedtime I fell asleep before the next cricket chirped. About midnight I suddenly awoke from a sound sleep. *Had something hit the camper, or was it a very loud knock on the door?*

My heart pounded rapidly as I sat up in bed.

"Blanche, I think there's someone outside!" I whispered. When I peeked out the side window I saw a hand holding what looked like a can. "Do you think it could be one of those spray cans whose contents temporarily blind you?"

Then came another loud knock. Finally I found my tongue. "Can I help you?"

"This is the rest stop attendant," said a voice. "You're parked crooked. There may be other people coming in later who might need parking space."

We thanked him and immediately reparked the van to his liking. We had parked on an angle to make our refrigerator as level as possible. It was a big relief that no one was breaking in.

We awoke the next morning to a partly cloudy sky, brisk winds from the north, and a temperature of 49°F. The cool air invigorated me, boosting my energy level over the top. Interstate 459 bypassed Birmingham, and I managed the heavy traffic on the alternate route without difficulty.

We left the freeway at 2:30 to visit Brakworth Elementary School in Birmingham. Once again I had the opportunity to talk to the children and teachers about choices, values, and attitudes. I told them how much these things determined whether or not my trip across America would be successful.

We later made another detour, this time onto State Route 65. This took us to Greater Birmingham Junior Academy, 20 miles out in the country. Built on top of a hill, the facility resembled an Eskimo village with each building shaped like a large igloo. The principal's residence was just below the hill, where Regina Vann, her husband, Ken, and their two children lived in a house that resembled a Spanish villa. The moment we entered the door we stepped back in time to the beginning of this century. Copper pots, tea kettles, frying pans, and copper molds of every size and shape hung from the kitchen rafters. Leaded glass graced the cupboard doors. An archway in an inside brick wall displayed spoons and glazed mugs and spices.

A shower is priceless when the dust and exhaust fumes from

the traffic have closed in on you all day. These folks, however, had an antique tub long enough and deep enough for me to lie back and completely relax in the warm water. After a leisurely bath it was off to bed around 10:00 to continue my dreams under a hand-crocheted bedspread.

The next morning we all piled into the Vanns' car and went downtown to Roebuck church. The school children presented a special program, and I enjoyed an opportunity to share a story from my childhood. It was a quiet, restful day. After supper we went back downtown to see the giant statue of Vulcan on top of Red Mountain. Vulcan, the mythical inventor of metalworking, represented the Roman god of fire. We rode the outside elevator to the top of the statue, then came down by the stairs—all 160 of them. I'm glad that I didn't have to depend on Vulcan to see me across America! We finally got to bed after 11:00.

Early the next morning Joan Smith, who taught at the academy, came by with her sister, Alice Vorrhus. They brought some pictures that the pastor of the Methodist church had developed for us. After a big breakfast, we went back to the church where the Pathfinder club was meeting in the assembly hall. Out came the black lung with the tumor in it. I doubt if any of the children will ever start smoking after seeing and hearing about the heart and lung I displayed for them. Afterward, all of us rode our bikes in formation before joining hands in a circle to pray for my safety on the road. What a great bunch of youngsters!

We were back on the freeway before noon. It took a while to locate the place where we had stopped on Friday because I had neglected to jot down the ramp number. I traveled a long, uphill grade just outside Birmingham, and guess what? I was back on that horrible shale again in heavy traffic on the freeway. But it wasn't really as bad as it sounds. The variety of trees along the roadside adorned themselves in lovely shades of green and yellow. Beautiful Logan-Martin Lake, with little islands in the middle, shimmered in the rays of the sun. We met caring people along the way, and I had the strength to keep going. So what more did we need?

Needed or not, I got more! R. L. Haynes, state trooper from

Jacksonville, stopped me to say I could not continue until his supervisor came by and talked to me. I agreed to meet them at the next off-ramp and gave him some newspaper clippings about our journey. My fervent prayers ascended heavenward.

As I walked along, pushing my bike across the rocky road at the truck stop, a nail made short work of my front tire. I spotted the auto repair sign a few yards away, and the attendant needed only minutes to fix the tire. Then Blanche and I prayed and waited. Finally, Trooper Haynes and his supervisor, Mark Williamson, arrived. Trooper Williamson had driven 40 miles to join us at the truck stop.

"If you made it safely through Mississippi," he said, "you'll do fine in Alabama. It's safer here. You may continue on your way."

By now it was 6:40. We had gone only two exits when the bike tire went flat again. Fortunately, Blanche was nearby. This time I asked the attendant to put in a new tube.

About 8:30 that night who should appear but the Vann family! I don't know how they found us. Ken wanted us to come back and spend the night again. Although touched by their thoughtfulness, I didn't think we should take the time to go back, only to have to return again in the morning. I needed to keep the wind to my back and my face to the rising sun.

When we crossed the border into Georgia, I was still in hilly country. The welcome center personnel greeted us and helped us get our bearings. About 65 school children came to the road to meet me. The underside of an overpass provided a perfect amphitheater for children and teachers to watch for me to come by. As bicycles do not usually travel on the interstate, they quickly recognized me as the person they wanted to see.

"Thanks to all of you for coming out to meet me," I began. "Many exciting things are happening in my life these days. So far nothing has stopped me from moving across America, one day at a time. Would you like to come with me?"

Most of them said they were afraid they would get too tired and couldn't keep going.

"It is important that you put much into life so that you can ex-

TO YOUR HEALTH!

It's time to add another letter from FRESH START! This time it's a "T" for The use of water. Water's great for drinking but has a lot of other uses as well. Of course it's important for keeping our clothes and bodies clean so that we don't reabsorb the poisons accumulating on the skin from the pores.

"The external application of water is one of the easiest and most satis-factory ways of regulating the circulation of the blood. A cold or cool bath is an excellent tonic. Warm baths open the pores and thus aid in the elim-ination of impurities. Both warm and neutral baths soothe the nerves and equalize the circulation" (Ministry of Healing, p. 237).

With inadequate water intake the blood itself becomes dehydrated and thickens. Reduced circulation by the thickened blood makes the brain an early and susceptible target. This is possibly one cause of senility, according to J. Carlton, Ph.D. Water is also the best liquid for cleansing the tissues.

Pure water, drunk some little time before or after a meal, is all that nature requires to quench thirst. Drinking a lot of liquid with meals di-lutes the gastric juices and delays digestion. Six to eight glasses of water a day will go a long way toward keeping sickness away from your door. Drink two glasses of warm water when you get up, two an hour before dinner, and two an hour before supper. (Clear the residual substances in the plumbing by letting the water run out of the tap a little before using it.) Do not depend on thirst to notify you it's time to take a drink. Some people never get thirsty. Dehydration can be a serious health hazard as well as cause you to not feel well. A sparkling glass of water can do won-ders for you.

pect to get much out of it," I told them. "Drifting carelessly with the tide just throws us back and forth against the beach. We miss all the adventure that helps us learn more and accomplish better things.

"Some of us are on a stationary bicycle. We never make the world around us very exciting because we aren't going anywhere. Each day, why don't you find someone who would feel better if you stopped to tell them that you appreciate something nice they do, and that you want to be their friend?

"Sometimes it is tough out here. Climbing steep hills, getting too much sun, all the noise on the freeway—these things make it hard to keep pedaling. But it's nice to know God cares about me and will help me reach my goals. You can choose to do the same. Hopefully, we can meet again sometime. I know you'll have a good report to give me then. Why don't we say a prayer before I start out again, asking God to take care of you here, and of me as I go down the road."

Channel 5 sent a crew to film me on the road. Everyone worked hard to make the story meaningful and interesting. Blanche and I even stayed up until 11:00 to watch the broadcast at a motel near the minimart where we had parked for the night.

A MOVIE IN ATLANTA

April 29. I had decided to visit nearby Madison, then return to Atlanta early on April 30 to meet the Thousand Oaks crew. We left milepost 61 in Atlanta and headed toward Madison. Several things delayed us on the road as we traveled. A couple on their way home to Augusta and two ladies who had seen us on TV stopped to chat. When a state patrolman stopped us, we took a picture of him standing by his patrol car.

Blanche arrived at the Madison exit about five minutes after I did. We went to a KOA and settled in to wash—us, our clothes, and the RV, inside and outside. The man camping next to us hooked up our sewage drain. The people who make up the U.S.A. have not lost their friendly touch! It's unfortunate that the world outside our borders often gets only the bad reports about us.

My meter recorded 52 miles for the day. About 11:00 we heard a plaintive call from geese flying overhead. Why hadn't they settled down on a lake somewhere for the night? Why wasn't *I* in bed asleep?

This was the big day! Blanche and I left the campground in the van at 7:00 and soon became part of the heavy morning traffic. We met Tim Patterson and his crew from Thousand Oaks at the Peachtree Inn in Atlanta. Tim brought us up to speed on what they hoped to accomplish in the next two days, and we worked out a schedule before they actually started filming.

First, they took pictures of Blanche and me inside the camper planning a typical day, talking about having everything ready to go, eating nourishing food, and studying the map to be sure we both understood where and when we would meet. Then I rode my bicycle down a hill that led to a main traffic artery entering town. The crew filmed shots from far above on the overpass, then close-up. Next they went ahead of me and took shots as I rode toward them. Then we were off to the country with the bike safely on the rack. A smooth road and open, restful countryside provided an excellent site for filming me riding the bike and racewalking along the shoulder.

This day, like so many others, seemed to come together so that we accomplished our goals. I had promised to speak to a group of nurses and staff at the Adventist hospital in Atlanta, as well as visit a local academy. These appointments gave the crew an opportunity to shoot footage of this aspect of my mission. The young people gathered in the courtyard with their teachers, willing to pose for the camera, and waited patiently while the crew adjusted the lighting and props. We had a fruitful day.

That evening the manager took us to the twelfth floor of the inn so we could look out over the city. The glitter of a million multicolored lights dazzled our eyes. It reminded me of the time I had climbed Grouse Mountain in British Columbia 50 years before and looked down on the lights below.

The next day was May Day, but we didn't spend it delivering May baskets. Instead, we worked with Tim and the crew until 3:00. They filmed us in the park eating by a lake, taking my bike off the rack, putting air in the tires, putting on gloves and helmet, adjusting the tape recorder and earphones, fixing the handlebar bag in place, filling my water bottle, snapping on the mileage meter, then doing a last-minute check before going out on the freeway once again. We finished the day with a shot of me relaxing on the grass in a park with the bicycle in the background.

Then Blanche and I were in the van and on our way back to Madison so I could resume my bike journey from the point I had stopped three days before. Before quitting for the day we went through Siloam and out the old highway to visit Frank Channelli and his family. Frank was superintendent of the main community schools in the area. We spent the night parked in their yard.

The next morning we headed toward Madison to attend

church. Along the way we stopped to have breakfast by a little pond. Cattle grazed in the fields. Flowers—sometimes a few, sometimes great gardens of them—bloomed along the way, and green pastures met the blue of the sky. What a nice day to put our cares aside and enjoy a restful change after our busy week!

We found the quaint, inviting church. Ethel Tolhurst, whom Gene and I had known while living in Japan, was there. Her husband had delivered Ladonna, our daughter. Church members invited us to have dinner with them. Our only problem was choosing from among the wonderful array of food.

That afternoon we visited Ethel's home, where she lived with her widower father. During a long walk across several fenced grasslands, we came upon a little house, unpainted and weathered with age, that had been built in 1941. To our delight, the woman who had come to the house as a bride 50 years before came through the pasture gate and walked over to talk with us. She remembered well those days of so long ago. There were few conveniences and some hardships, but happy times as well.

Later Ethel took us downtown to see some of the restored old homes and mansions. Afterward we said goodbye and headed back to Siloam. The Channellies, our hospitable host and hostess, were still up and waiting for us. Once again we spent the night in their yard.

The bike's wheels were in motion by 8:10 next morning. We rode along Interstate 20, hoping to cross the border between Georgia and South Carolina before dark. Then we would be on the last lap of the journey. An excellent shoulder helped me to cover the miles quickly—42 of them by noon! Even though there were hills, hills, and more hills, my muscles proved adequate to the task.

We ate dinner outdoors at a rest stop. Evelyn Mead, an 81-years-young lady who was traveling alone, stopped to visit with us as we ate. Looking at her, I was reminded once more that it's not years but choices that determine what we can do and when. In Hunza Land, high in the mountains of India, the older one gets the wiser he or she becomes. In that place old age does not dictate when one must stop climbing the steep hills to work in the fields.

The rich mineral water from the mountains, homegrown food, exercise, and a relaxed schedule all help to prevent cancer, coronaries, and other degenerative diseases. Some areas have no doctors, no modern medical wonders, no up-to-the-minute equipment, and few medicines. When it's time to die, sometimes after a century or more, the old person often simply slips away quietly.

Back on the road again after dinner, we were stopped by an ambulance with two attendants. When they waved to me I stopped to speak with them. "We heard your story on the media. Is there anything we can do to help you?" one of them asked. "Is there anything you need?"

One young man handed me two compresses. "These can be activated by breaking a capsule inside which sets up a reaction, making the compress very cold. It's good for sprains or other injuries," he explained.

FINISHED AT LAST

I called Gene Jr. for the last time before we would see him in Charleston. He was recovering from a bout with the flu but planned to leave the next day and meet us just outside Charleston. He would set things up for the grand finale. Gene Sr. told me he was counting the days until we returned home to Michigan.

Highway 78 toward Charleston looked like the best route to take. I biked through Aiken that has a population of 15,000 people and more than 900 thoroughbred horses that wintered there. The terrain, sandy roads, and mild climate made it an ideal sports ground. It was here I met Sissy Brodie. Sissy saw me on the street and introduced herself. She belonged to a cycle club she actively promoted. She went to the newspaper office to let them know about our arrival, but the office was empty. So she used some of our film to take photographs to give to the newspaper and promised to send the negatives to Gene.

As we said goodbye to Sissy, a teacher from Mead Hall Episcopal School spotted us. "Please come and speak to our fourth through sixth graders, will you?" she asked.

TO YOUR HEALTH!

It's time to talk a little about the "A" in FRESH START. This letter stands for Abstemiousness. What a word! Abstain. What if we all used this key every time we made a choice? We would eat just the right amount of the right things. No one would need to depend on alcohol, tobacco, coffee, or other drugs. We would all get enough exercise and rest and drink plenty of water. There wouldn't be a sick person among us!

Alcohol causes aggregation of cells and can destroy brain cells. Bone loss (a form of osteoporosis) may be due in part to the direct effects of ethanol. Studies link caffeinated beverages, such as coffee and soft drinks, with breast cysts, bladder disease, pancreas disease, and much of the anxiety and nervousness people experience today. Smoking is the greatest preventable risk factor and causes the largest amount of sickness and death in America today.

Because the will holds in check unhealthful or unacceptable habits, new correct habit pathways can be laid down and strengthened by frequent repetition. Inhibitory nerve pathways to the unacceptable old habits can be formed. Everything depends on the use of the will (see Ministry of Healing, p. 176).

If we give our will to Christ He will work it all out for us. More studies are showing that body, mind, and soul must work together for lasting results. Overworking, overeating, overexcitement—all the "overs"—are harmful. Balance is the key.

White letters on a large blue sign announced "South Carolina Welcomes You." I felt a twinge of sadness as we crossed the last border. From California to South Carolina I had experienced changes in weather, terrain, flora, soil, lakes, and people. I wondered if I had changed as they changed. Was there more love in my heart for those who had to work hard to make a living, in spite of poor soil and harsh elements? What about those whose homes nestled in the mountains, surrounded by lakes and wild flowers and everything one needs to be happy? Peace and contentment, I had discovered, must come from within ourselves. Our own attitudes and love for God and our fellow humans determine whether or not we have the inner peace that the world cannot take away.

We had to be in Charleston by the 7th. I hated to disappoint her, though, and—you guessed it—shortly afterward arrived at the school. Once more, out came the human heart and lungs.

By 2:00 we were back on the road again. I pedaled through pecan groves and woods, and beside tobacco fields. We stopped at a roadside vegetable and fruit market in Denmark. The folks there insisted on giving us two boxes of strawberries. We also bought a watermelon, red bell peppers, and other goodies. At supper that night I ate a whole box of strawberries!

We decided to stay in a Hardee's parking lot for the night. Although heavy rain fell throughout the evening, we were dry and warm. After Hardee's closed for the night, a fight broke out near the restaurant. We wondered whether we should remain parked there, but the disturbance ended in a few minutes.

We awoke on May 5 realizing we would enter Charleston that day. An overcast sky and a whirling wind promised a dismal day ahead. A warm breakfast at Hardee's sounded good to me, so off we went, where we met two wildlife and marine officers who were also having breakfast. When I asked them for the best way out of town and into Charleston, they suggested Route 61 through Bamberg.

Blanche arrived at a quaint little town first and stopped to mail letters and find the press. When I arrived at the van, Betty Whitehouse from a nearby florist shop beckoned me inside. A former nurse, she had just received her master florist degree. We enjoyed a brief visit before I left. She caught up with me several miles down the road and handed me two red roses. I hugged her and thanked her for coming so far to bring the roses to me. Blanche later told me what had happened.

"Betty got so excited that she called the newspaper and then jumped in her car and headed east to try and find you on the road."

Real love and friendship don't come in colors, customs, or creeds—just in hearts beating together in unison. I will never forget those two red roses or the new friend who brought them to me.

With the wind behind me, I made good time. We stopped briefly in Canady, where Blanche took a walk and discovered the large Canady family cemetery. While picking up some propane gas that we used for cooking and running the refrigerator, she learned that the attendant at the shop had a rare liver disease. He told her he had opened his small bait and bar shop to get away from the noise and confusion of the "big town." One thing in particular interested Blanche.

"He had only lower teeth," she remarked, "and his wife had only uppers."

Time to eat. Food was a welcome sight after five hours on the road. We had just finished eating when we heard a knock.

"Is someone hurt?" asked the gentleman outside the door.

Pastor Veronee from the nearby Baptist church had noticed my bike lying in the grass and was worried. This pastor obviously liked people. During our short visit we learned that his parish had doubled in size since his arrival.

When we took to the road again, we were still about 24 miles from Charleston. I passed a family with seven children waiting at the side of the road.

"We belong to Pastor Veronee's church," they told me when I stopped, "and we wanted to meet you and wish you well."

I was almost to Charleston. The time had come to call a halt to any more motion for the day. We stopped at a fire lookout station. "Would you mind if we parked up near the lookout station for the night?" I asked the family who lived on the property.

"We'd be happy to have you park there," the woman responded, "but we have 29 hound dogs who bark at every little commotion within earshot."

As I needed to be wide awake the next day to ride through Charleston, we decided to look elsewhere. Pastor Veronee called his father and received permission for us to stop overnight at fire station number three. So we headed for Charleston.

Chief Veronee, his navy-blue uniform resplendent with gold braid, welcomed us. "Well, I have never had women as guests here overnight before, but we want to welcome you," he told us.

The night crew hooked up our camper, and the boys at the station stayed in the parlor watching TV while we took over the bathroom. We enjoyed a good night's sleep away from the busy highway.

As I mentioned earlier, my son, Gene, planned to meet us in Charleston. Unfortunately, due to a mix-up, I had the name of the wrong hotel. When he wasn't there, I called several other possible hotels, but no Gene. The airport couldn't trace him, and I had no idea where to find him. There is a Bible promise that says if with a humble heart we seek God's help in every need He will guide us as to the best course to take. My decision for the moment was to go to bed and get a good rest. I could have stayed awake through the night worrying, but I chose to put my concern in the hands of One who knew all along where Gene was and would surely direct him to where we were.

When we got up early the next morning, the coldness of night still hung in the air as the sun made its appearance. Pastor Veronee, bless him, stopped by to see if all was well. Once more I tried to trace Gene, but still had no word from him. I needed to hurry back to the home of the baying hounds and resume my ride from where I had stopped the night before. I was inside the camper getting ready to leave when I heard a deep, radio-announcer-type voice with the volume turned up, talking to Blanche outside. Gene had found us! If we had parked by the Middelton Inn he probably would not have seen us because of the trees. We could have been on Highway 78, or even 26, the main freeway into Charleston—but here we were! And to think that he arrived almost to the minute before I left to ride back to Charleston. I got a big hug, which helped to dissolve some of the loneliness of the long hours out on the road.

When I left, Gene was already at work contacting the media. Forgetting everything else, I put my best efforts into closing the gap between the Atlantic Ocean and myself. And I made it into Charleston before Gene did! People driving to work during the morning rush hour saw the ACROSS AMERICA sign around my waist and cooperated beautifully by giving me space on the shoulderless road. Many motorists honked their horns in welcome, seeming to know that this was "the end of the trail" for me. Suddenly I looked up—and into the camera of WCBD-TV. A cameraman sat on the vehicle's tailgate, filming me as I rode along.

When I reached the fire station, Gene and I reenacted our welcoming hug for the TV camera. Pastor Veronee came by again with his wife and several other friends. They sang a song for us and offered their help in any way. Before I left the fire station I received strict instructions not to go down to the beach that day to officially end my trip. I must wait until the mayor and other officials could accompany me in the morning.

Once more I rode alone, searching my way across the city toward Folly Beach, where I would meet the mayor the next day. I stopped along the way at O Bikeway Cycle Center, a Schwinn bicycle shop. It took the friendly young owner only about 10 minutes to put my bike up on the rack and give it a quick inspection. He refused any payment for his work and gave me a nice water bottle with his shop's name on the outside. I shall take good care of it and will always treasure the memory of his buoyant spirit.

A newspaper reporter from Charleston stopped me at the side of the road. He had looked for me earlier and missed me. I explained why I couldn't go to the beach until the next day, so he got his picture and information and headed back to the city. I stopped at Pelican Cove, an RV campground near the ocean. They placed a lovely bouquet in my arms and invited us to hook up and be their guests for the night.

A little farther down the road a sign in front of the Holiday Inn proclaimed, "Welcome, Mrs. Hamlin!" Barry Shield, the manager, was out talking to Blanche when I arrived and invited us to stay at the inn as their guests. I felt that we should accept the first invitation from Pelican Cove for that night. However, we did accept the inn's invitation for the following two nights.

TO YOUR HEALTH!

"R," the next-to-last letter in FRESH START, *stands for* **Restoration.** *The Bible says, "'But I will restore you to health and heal your wounds,' declares the Lord" (Jer. 30:17, NIV).*

"The burden of disease and wretchedness and sin He came to remove. It was His mission to bring to men complete restoration; He came to give them health and peace and perfection of character.

"Varied were the circumstances and needs of those who besought His aid, and none who came to Him went away unhelped. From Him flowed a stream of healing power, and in body and mind and soul men were made whole" (**Ministry of Healing**, *p. 17*).

Curt Norman, a photographer from United Press International, arrived to take pictures. Before we finished he had me out on the sharp, slippery boulders of the breakwater. I fell and received a few superficial wounds. Curt felt badly, but all of my bones were intact and the helmet had protected my head.

For the next picture Curt handed me a piece of cake. With my bicycle propped up in the foreground I raised my left arm with cake in hand, high over my head. Two gulls immediately came to share the spotlight with me! In the 8½ x 11 photograph Curt later sent us it looked as if the gulls and I were enjoying the greatest adventure life had to offer. The joy of having finished a task I had set out to accomplish radiated from my upturned face. Curt's ability to use the incoming waves against the breakwater, the gulls in flight, and the ocean stretching far away showed great talent. I shall always cherish that picture. In his accompanying letter Curt wrote, "I hope that you have seen this picture previously in one of UPI's member papers. I do recall that I received *very* favorable comments when I transmitted it, so there is a great chance that it received good play. I was amazed when I saw my picture with you in one of the publications that you sent! What an honor!

"I do hope that all continues to go well with you. I wish that I had more contact with you so that some of your healthy habits could rub off on me!"

Back at the cove that evening everyone enjoyed watching the pelicans as they swooped, circled, and rode on the air currents above the hotel. On the other side of the hotel a high terrace rose above the retaining wall, where the waves sent great clouds of spray into the air. Tomorrow I would walk down those steps beside the wall and into the Atlantic Ocean to officially mark the end of my journey. As I crawled into bed for the last time before the big day we had for so many months hoped and prayed would arrive, I felt a little guilty. I had already been down on the breakwater—Curt had eased me out onto that beach. Well, I still hadn't gone down *into* the ocean.

I awoke next morning with the realization that my journey was almost finished. In spite of the excitement, I suffered a sense of loss of time and space and freedom. Soon I would return to the responsibility of helping others choose a lifestyle that would put assets in the bank of health, rather than remove them: I decided to look at that assignment as just the continuation of what I was already doing.

Tom Marshall, acting chief of the Folly Beach Public Safety Department, arrived to escort us to the Holiday Inn. At the inn we would proceed onto the deck for the ceremony. The mayor, Dr. Richard Beck, members of his staff, and city council members joined me for the last 500 yards. Burt and Louise Elkins, who had been members of my Walla Walla College graduating class 48 years before, appeared from nowhere at the last minute! A group of schoolchildren from a nearby Christian school joined us. A pastor came and offered a lovely prayer, thanking God for my safety and for helping me in so many ways to make it to the finish.

A swimming pool, its water sparkling blue and calm in the morning sunlight, added a pleasant touch to the deck. Dr. Beck gave a short speech filled with complimentary remarks. Someone placed a large bouquet of red roses in my arms. I thanked everyone for their contributions in making this day such a memorable one. Then I removed my watch, shoes, helmet, and glasses and, accompanied by Gene, walked down the steps to the water. I ran back and forth through the surf as cameras recorded the event.

It was over. I had completed my journey.

HOMEWARD BOUND

We spent several days in New York at the headquarters for the van ministries blood pressure screening program. In this program young people go out in specially equipped buses to screen people for blood pressure problems. They encourage clients to change their lifestyles to improve their bodies, minds, and souls. Some of the drivers and attendants are former drug addicts, smokers, or alcoholics. Every day van personnel find someone who needs help in some way. One may be contemplating suicide, another to kill somebody, a third to give up trying. Be they government officials, the rich and the famous, or the beggar on the street, the ministries workers treat and help everyone.

One morning we met Mayor Koch of New York City. Our

group included Blanche and Pastor Kretchmar, then president of the Greater New York Conference of Seventh-day Adventists. Juanita, his wife, is the founder of the van ministries. At city hall we sat on a bench and waited while a receptionist, stationed between us and the mayor's office, kept us posted as to what we should do and when. Finally the mayor, flanked by five bodyguards, came through the door.

"Where did you go?" asked Mayor Koch.

"I went from Oceanside, California, to Charleston, South Carolina."

"Now she wants to go across Europe," Pastor Kretchmar told him.

"Why not come with me?" I invited the mayor.

"Tell me where you'll be and I'll come!" he laughed. Then the mayor asked me to put on my helmet while pictures were taken.

We all appreciated the time he gave us from his busy schedule. Now it was time to go home. Even though Blanche is a good driver, I decided to get behind the wheel myself as we drove out of New York and into Pennsylvania. I enjoyed the challenge, but I must admit that I breathed a sigh of relief as we finally left the city behind us.

Our next stop was Lansing, Michigan, to meet Lieutenant Governor Martha W. Griffiths at the capitol. What to wear? I didn't have a lot of up-to-the-minute clothes in my wardrobe, but I'm not one to stay awake worrying about such things. Things usually fall into place when the time comes. I did have a pink-and-gray warm-up suit that I had received as a gift back in 1978. So I wore the warm-up suit jacket and touring bicycle shorts that had big pockets on the sides. The ACROSS AMERICA sign wrapped around my waist finished off my ensemble. This was really more representative of what I was doing than a dress or suit.

Lieutenant Governor Griffiths presented me with a framed certificate of appreciation from Michigan governor James Blanchard that read: "To Charlotte Hamlin, for your contributions as assistant professor of nursing and coordinator of the Fresh Start program at Andrews University. Your 2,500-mile 'Walk Across America,' the purpose of which is to show older people what can be accomplished if they stay active following retirement, is certainly inspiring."

Senator Harry Gast, Representatives Lad Stacey and Carl Gnodtke from Districts 44 and 43 in our area, and Olivia Maynard, director, Office of Aging, state of Michigan, also attended the presentation.

We arrived back home in a drizzling rain on the morning of May 20. Gene Sr. was the first in line for a big hug. I so much appreciated the mail he had sent during my travels, and I was so glad he was there for the homecoming.

Gene Jr. had the morning's events scheduled down to the minute. We started our procession from a parking lot in "downtown" Berrien Springs. I received a hug from the police chief while the newspaper reporter took our picture. At 10:30 we left the parking lot, with Blanche driving behind me for the last time. She is a great scout and true friend. I will never forget all that she did to make the trip successful. We traveled about a mile before turning into Apple Valley Plaza. Excitement ran high as the band played ahead of me. A young man, Beau Shine, walked beside me, pushing my bicycle. He represented children everywhere who are building healthy bodies while young. I had met many like him out on the road.

Dr. Lesher, then president of Andrews University, welcomed me home. The senior pastor of Pioneer Memorial church, where I had been a member for many years, offered a prayer of thanksgiving for my safe return. The Nursing Department presented me with red roses. President Moon of Berrien Springs gave me a key to the city. Apple Valley Market provided a large cake, shaped like the United States, that showed my route from beginning to end, even including the states' borders and the mountain ranges.

I spoke to the group for a few minutes, thanking them for their prayers. I thanked the press for their interest in my venture, and an interview with a journalist from Detroit marked the end of the occasion. The next day I was back in my office.

TO YOUR HEALTH!

And now for the last letter in FRESH START, the last "T." It stands for Trust in divine power.

Our life is a triangle, made up of three components: physical, mental, and spiritual. Remove any one of the three sides and the structure collapses. We also have three sections in our brain. Any one of them can have a lot to do with the choices we make all through life. Toward the back of our brain is the intellect center, housing memory, sight, and hearing. The motor area, where touch and control of muscle movements take place, covers the center of the brain. The third section is the frontal lobe, where we develop our thinking, personality, and character. We also develop our moral and spiritual values and beliefs in this great powerhouse.

What does all this mean? A person may have one highly developed area, or perhaps lack development in one area. For example, one may not have any sense of morality, mercy, or justice, or the ability to sympathize, but may have a computer-like ability to remember numbers. Most education today does not teach on a spiritual level, but develops only the intellectual and motor areas. For this reason many young people view life as a battle of wits. Some choose not to make a choice on values, religion, or beliefs. Some lack motivation to do anything. When the frontal lobe is underdeveloped, a person operates on the pleasure principle from the motor area, the location of touch and control of muscle movements. (From the article "Living Body," Life and Health.)

"[The will] . . . is the governing power in the nature of man—the power of decision, of choice. Everything depends on the right action of the will" (Ministry of Healing, p. 176).

If we choose to serve God and give Him our will, our whole nature will come under His control, putting Him in charge of the decisions we must make.

An extensive study of smokers who have gone through the Five-Day Plan to Stop Smoking reveals that 25 percent have remained smoke-free. These are the ones who felt it was not right for them to smoke and that they needed God's help in order to remain smoke-free. This same power accompanied me across this continent and brought me safely back home. God will do great things for those who put their trust in Him.

FRESH START: Fresh air, Rest, Exercise, Simple diet, Happiness, Sunshine, The use of water, Abstemiousness, Restoration, and Trust in divine power. Make these principles part of your life. They will help you find the lifestyle that will set you free!

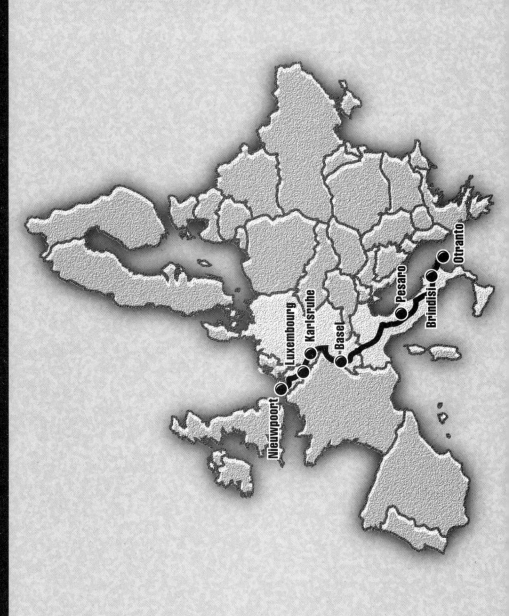

Nieuwpoort

Luxembourg

Karlsruhe

Basel

Pesaro

Brindisi

Otranto

OFF TO EUROPE

On a beautiful fall day I officially cleared out a 15-year accumulation from my office in the Department of Nursing at Andrews University. The time had come for my trip to Europe.

On September 2, 1987, Cecilia Seabury, who would be my driver, and I left from Chicago's O'Hare International Airport for Luxembourg, a small country tucked between Belgium and Germany. When Cecilia and I had first met at a health fair in Berrien Springs, she asked if she could ride with me through Europe.

"Sure, why not," I'd replied.

Unfortunately, she developed a problem with her knees while riding her bike to prepare for our trip. When I told her what I really needed was a driver for my support vehicle, she immediately volunteered for the job.

Bad news awaited us when my bicycle was unloaded in Luxembourg. The bicycle had received some damage to the brakes in transit. I wondered if this would prove hazardous as I rode through the mountains. In the end I decided that we'd do our best; things would work out OK. So we loaded the bike and ourselves into a Hertz rental car, and by 7:30 p.m. we were on our way to the coast of Belgium.

In Brussels we passed by a large street carnival in full swing. It looked like fun, but we didn't take time to stop. About midnight we stopped at the little village of Nieuwpoort for a glass of grape juice. Even at that hour, the small bar at Trinity Hotel still had many customers. The proprietor recommended the Pacific Hotel on the next block for our overnight stop. The hotel, presided over by a chubby, sleepy-eyed owner, looked like something from a storybook. Our weary bodies welcomed the opportunity to completely relax, and we slept soundly.

The next morning's continental breakfast in the dining room consisted of large rolls in a basket, butter, cheese, jam, and cocoa, served on white tablecloths, starched and ironed to perfection. After breakfast Cecilia went downtown to meet Etienne De Salver, director of tourism. He presented her with two pewter plates and two toilet kits as gifts from the city. We returned later and had our picture taken with Mr. De Salver on the steps outside his office. Two nice-looking young gentlemen, Leo Bonte and Ian Huyghe, interviewed us that afternoon, then took us down to the Nieuwpoort Beach boardwalk and pier. At a bike shop near the beach an attendant checked the damaged brakes on my bicycle and did what he could to repair them. They were somewhat better when he finished working on them.

That evening the city gave us a complimentary meal at the Pacific Hotel. The hotel personnel did everything they could to make the dinner a memorable experience. By the time we finished the numerous courses, we thought a walk around town for exercise would be a good idea. We finally got to bed late, tired, but happy.

As usual, Saturday was my day off. We visited the O. L. Vroowkerk Cathedral near the square. Built in 1163, the Gothic building had been restored after suffering damage in World War II. On March 20, 1939, Leopold the Third declared it to be a classified monument. Its stained glass windows, ornate carvings, and artwork are priceless reminders of an era when people took the time to mold their talents into permanent treasures. Near the altar sat a replica of a ship that had disappeared in a 1986 storm while crossing the channel to England. Only one person, a 15-year-old boy from Nieuwpoort, survived.

In the countryside small herds of cattle and sheep grazed in the fields near houses of brick and ceramic tile, or block and stucco. Beautiful lace curtains danced at the windows in the gentle breeze above window boxes spilling over with colorful flowers.

About 10 kilometers from Nieuwpoort we visited the site where 250,000 English soldiers had died in World War I, one of more than 140 military cemeteries in the area. The Belgians donated—and still maintain—the cemetery area in nearby Roesolere. As we looked across fields covered with rows of white markers, a heavy rain began to fall. How the tears must have fallen like rain in thousands of homes where a boy would never again bound up the front steps announcing, "I'm home!" Wherever we went, people remembered and were thankful for the great sacrifice the people of the United States had made on their behalf.

I had originally planned to start from Normandy Beach the next morning, but it was quite a distance north of Nieuwpoort. I decided to use Nieuwpoort as my point of departure. Cecilia and I made a last stop at the bike shop. Then my wheels and I once more faced life together as we began a trek that would take us across Belgium, through Luxembourg, over the hills of Germany, down the Rhine River, across the Swiss Alps, through the plains of northern Italy, and beside the Adriatic Sea to the last city in the heel of Italy's "boot."

We planned to go through Diksmuide first, then branch off to Roeselare. Cecilia would drive the rental car to Munich, where we planned to pick up a camper. As I had done on my trip across the United States a few months earlier, if I had to fill my water bottle or take care of other needs, I would leave the bike close to the road where Cecilia could see it. We agreed that if I passed our car and Cecilia wasn't in it (or perhaps was asleep), I would tuck a piece of red yarn under the windshield wiper to let her know I had passed her.

I knew I would meet people of different cultures and dialects and would somehow have to find a way to communicate with them. And I would have to deal with exchanging money in each country. In spite of all the possible obstacles, I was filled with excitement as I began my journey.

Cecilia passed me in Roeselare about 4:35 p.m., and then went on ahead to buy groceries. By 7:45 it was dark and raining. It took a while, but we did locate each other and stopped at the home of a Flemish couple to ask if they knew where we might find accommodations for the night. We left the bike there and drove to the little village of Kooigen, where we met Mrs. Henriette Defever-Vandevoorde. Henriette directed us to a building where we could spend the night. From the look of it, it had been vacant for some time. The place was quite dirty and had a gaping hole in the back door where someone had evidently broken in at some point.

We discovered a hanging cord which, when connected to power, produced running cold water. Henriette brought us some cots and sleeping bags and invited us to have breakfast with her and her husband the next morning. Then she was gone, and we were left to the cold, damp reality of life.

When we arrived at Henriette's home the next morning I could see why it would be risky to invite strangers into their home. She operated the village bank from her front room! It wasn't long until people began to arrive to do business. Henriette was still in her housecoat, but no one seemed to mind. As we ate our rolls, jam, and cheese, I realized the effort that Henriette had put forth to be hospitable and helpful to us.

Back on the road, Cecilia and I discovered it wasn't easy to keep track of each other. From Kortrijk we had taken N50 to Tournai. This definitely was not like the interstate system back home. However, I used the alternate routes that ran fairly close to the autobahn and moved along beautifully.

Cecilia drove ahead to Tournai to wait for me. When I didn't arrive, she went to the police station. They were very hospitable and gave her key rings for each of us with a logo of the world on it. She finally drove on to Beaumont, arriving there at 6:00 p.m. Then there was nothing to do but wait—and wonder where I was.

While it took her less than an hour to go 60 miles, it took me nearly all day to go that distance on my bike. I rode in the dark until 11:00. It was cool and the riding was easy, but because I couldn't see the road very well I drove into a ditch. Fortunately, I wasn't hurt.

By the time Cecilia got to town the police were off duty for the night, and the office closed. She reached them by telephone, but no one had seen me. Finally she decided to drive back a few miles to see if she could find me. There I was, soaked to the skin, pushing my bike along on the side of the road. We shared a mutual feeling of relief at the sight of each other and realized we had to find a better way to keep in touch on those narrow roads and still allow Cecilia to keep up with the flow of traffic.

We needed to find a place to spend the night. *Would anything be open at that late hour?* I wondered. As usual, I prayed. I saw a dim light in an unusual-looking building and could see someone walking around inside. We knocked on the rustic, hand-hewn door and explained our situation to the gentleman who answered. The building housed a restaurant and hotel, and we soon had a room for the night. All the plumbing and wiring in this interesting establishment was exposed on the foot-thick whitewashed walls. Even though we managed to get only lukewarm water for the enormous old tub, it helped to remove the day's accumulated grime.

The next morning the proprietor had breakfast waiting for us in the dining room. We learned the building was a converted barn, and our breakfast was served next to the manger where animals had once munched their hay.

After breakfast we picked up the bicycle and ran some errands. Few people could speak English, but we managed to communicate. It was afternoon by the time we resumed our journey. Unfortunately, I started out too soon after eating, and something I had eaten made my stomach feel a little squeamish. The heat of the sun added to my discomfort. I decided to go into a little town and look for an ice-cream cone to soothe my stomach and neutralize whatever was causing my discomfort. Well, to be honest, I think I mostly wanted an ice-cream cone.

Cecilia, not realizing that I had left the road, passed by while I was in the town. The road took her through a very dark forest on a lonely section of the road. She wished we were traveling this section together. It was one of the few areas where she felt a woman should not travel alone. She arrived in Neufchâteau 6:15 and bought some food while she waited for me to arrive, not realizing she was almost a day's journey ahead of me! When I hadn't arrived by 11:00, she checked into Terminus Hotel and trusted God to take care of me.

In the meantime I returned to the road after finishing my ice cream. It wasn't long until I also passed through the dark woods, miles from anywhere, and darkness began to overtake me. Strangely, I wasn't afraid. When I arrived in Beauraing, I realized I needed to find a place to sleep and would have to wait until morning to try to locate Cecilia. At a cafe-hotel I asked about lodging for the night. The owner looked at me, a white-haired, 68-year-old woman dragging a bike, wearing touring shorts and a bicycle helmet—and wearing grease from the bicycle chain on the calf of my right leg.

"Everything is closed; you can't find a room," he said. "There is a larger hotel several blocks over. Maybe you could try there."

I left my bike and a copy of a German newspaper article about my trip at the cafe and set out to look for the other hotel. By the time I returned, the owner's attitude had changed.

"We want you to stay right here with us and have dinner," he said.

After the cafe closed at 10:00 I enjoyed sitting around the kitchen table with the family for a meal of meat, fried potatoes, and vegetables. They seemed concerned that I didn't eat meat, and I wasn't sure they understood my explanation about being a vegetarian. After supper I retired to a lovely room upstairs and fell asleep, trusting that my driver and friend was safe and warm in bed somewhere.

The next morning Cecilia and I both awakened with the same question: "Where is she?" I thanked my hosts for the overnight accommodations (for which they refused to accept any payment). As I was looking around wondering what to do next, I found a gentleman who spoke English. What a blessing! Michael Brack had trained in Los Angeles as a chiropractor. He invited me to his home several blocks away where he asked his wife, Claudine, to help me find Cecilia. Claudine took me to the police station, and it wasn't long before Cecilia and I were talking to each other on the telephone. We agreed that Cecilia would wait in Neufchâteau.

I got there that evening about 6:00, pushing my bike up the

hill into town. Cecilia had bought some food and taken it to her room at the small hotel. The tomato sandwiches and fruit tasted wonderful! We both stayed at the hotel that night. How much better it would have been if I had not followed my nose into that village off the road the previous day.

The next day, September 10, I decided that Cecilia should go on alone to Frankfurt, turn in the car, and finalize a contract on a camper. While she waited for me to arrive she could visit with friends and relatives there and in Munich. She had married a G.I. during World War II and come to America as a war bride when she was 16. I put a few clothes in the carrier on the bicycle. Cecilia and I said a prayer together in front of the Terminus Hotel. We hugged each other and shed a few tears as we said goodbye; then I turned my cycle toward Highway N 85 and Bastogne.

Once again I was alone, just as I'd been for 10 days going across America. God had taken care of me before, and I knew He would now. Of course, I couldn't read the signs, understand the people, or count out the right change, but the unknown wouldn't stay that way very long. The roads were good and the weather pleasant. As I climbed higher into the hills the air became cooler. I loved it! Then, somehow, I got onto the autobahn. It was smooth on the shoulder, and I certainly made some fast time until two patrolmen came along and stopped me. They wanted to know what I was doing on the autobahn.

"This is where a man down the road instructed me to go," I told them.

They were very cordial, but showed me how to get off and find the alternate route at the top of the off-ramp. When I reached the road in the little town, a man got out of his car and came toward me. I had never had a stranger become so angry with me before. "Are you trying to kill yourself?" he roared. "Why were you down on the autobahn? Can't you read signs?"

With a big smile on my face, I tapped him on the shoulder and asked him to wait a minute and let me explain. At first I could only get a word in here and there as he continued to berate me. He finally calmed down when he understood that I had received the wrong directions and had no intention of committing suicide out on the autobahn. When I explained the purpose of my ride, he ended up driving miles out of his way to be sure that I stayed on the right road to reach the alternate route.

At Hotel ZurPfalz I received a complimentary meal with all the trimmings. It seemed that when I was alone on the road I met more people, heard more interesting stories, and received invitations into more inner circles than when I had a support van. Basically, human beings are protective, caring creatures.

I spent more than an hour in the city center of Bastogne, looking at the tanks and other reminders of World War II. Everyone seemed happy to meet an American tourist. Between Bastogne and Luxembourg some folks from the Netherlands stopped to get my picture and address. They signed their name as "Fam, A. J. Nykamp." They spoke English quite well and were ready to help in any way they could with directions and information.

At a cemetery outside Luxembourg thousands of white crosses stood in perfect rows, marking the final resting place for World War II soldiers. An immense memorial with the U.S. Army insignia stood in front of the crosses. A deep silence permeated the whole area. While there I met Steve Yates and his wife from the American Embassy in Paris. Together we experienced a feeling of sadness, mingled with pride, for the sacrifice represented by the crosses. Someday soon the great General of all time shall return, as He has promised, and call forth from those resting places the ones who loved and honored Him.

I arrived in Mersch and registered at an inexpensive hotel. I had left Nieuwpoort Beach on the coast of Belgium on September 6 and made it almost back to Luxembourg by the 11th. As I prepared for a quiet day off the road I could sense the unseen Guide directing me and seeing that my needs were met along the way. More than anything else I appreciated my safe passage through villages and on the roads. One advantage of traveling alone is that I couldn't lose anybody but myself. However, there were disadvantages—no one to cook healthy meals and have them ready when needed, no place to enjoy a short siesta after lunch, no place to change into dry clothes if it rained, and no ready-made place to sleep at night. Also, the extra baggage on the bike produced more wind resistance, requiring more energy to get over the hills. Most of all, though, I missed Cecilia. I had no one to laugh with.

MY FIRST CRASH

I didn't have a visa for France, so I planned to go through western Germany and down beside the Rhine River. When I showed people the route, they just shook their heads. It wasn't long until I found out why. My choice took me through mountains where I had to walk, pushing my bike. Coasting down the other side helped to even things out a little. I decided that the lush evergreens, beautiful gorges, and peaceful hillsides in many shades of green were worth the extra effort.

Most of the villages were located in valleys. One day as I approached a village, trying to watch the road signs, I ran into the curb at the bottom of a hill and lost control of the bike. I had been moving at a good clip, and the right side of my body took a real jolt when I landed. My helmet probably saved my life, because my head hit the sidewalk with a bang as my body skidded along the sidewalk. In seconds the rough cement scraped away the skin from my right arm and upper thigh. Big drops of blood formed on my right forearm but, fortunately, I didn't break any bones.

My first thought was to see if my cycle had been damaged. I didn't know what I'd do if the accident had broken some irreplaceable part. A close inspection revealed that the right lever controlling some of the gears had turned backward, but everything else seemed to have survived the impact. Not knowing what else to do, I took some food from the box on my bike and sat down to eat lunch. After eating, I walked across the street. A passing carload of people stared at me, apparently horrified by my condition. Several of them spoke at once in a language I didn't understand, then someone rounded up a few Band-Aids which they pressed into my hand before speeding away.

A young man saw me walking slowly along the street and came

to my assistance. "You come with me," he said in English. "I will take care of you."

He took me to his apartment where I met his wife. Danielle and Claude Branco-Weber offered me food and assistance with my injuries. As he cleaned my wounds and covered them with bandages, Claude told me I was in Sandweiler, Luxembourg. Before I left, Preve Schlmitt, the mayor, took a picture of the three of us on the steps of the building. Back on the road once more, I covered many miles before dusk. I was sore the next day but still managed to cover 53 miles.

Going through the city of Luxembourg provided a real challenge. I had no idea whether to start into the city or to go around. Monique Winter, a lovely lady I met on the street, came to my rescue. According to her business card, she lived at Grand Duchy of Luxembourg. She certainly seemed like a Grand Duchess in my book. That dear lady drove ahead of me for miles. We went around corners, down one street and up another until we came safely out on the other side of Luxembourg.

As I rode along the road, relaxed and enjoying the scenery, I experienced a deep feeling of gratitude toward God, who had created all the beauty around me. It felt good to be alive. Once again the road took me through dense forests. I wondered whether I would find overnight accommodations before dark in this sparsely populated countryside. When I stopped to eat at a little roadside cafe I met Tlanuela and Gerhard Hauser, who were touring on a motorbike. A little later I was on my way again, traveling east, when the Hausers came up beside me on their bike and offered to take me to an inn a short distance down the road. Gerhard went on ahead on the motorbike to make reservations, while Tlanuela and I walked to the inn, with me pushing my bicycle. Their help meant a lot. I was not looking forward to spending a night in the woods.

Riding through Pirmasens the next day I came upon a huge U.S. Army installation. I was allowed to enter the base but couldn't eat in the mess hall; civilians were not admitted. I decided to forgo the greasy food at the little concession stand in favor of some of the food I had with me. I enjoyed the opportunity to visit with some of the enlisted personnel; one girl even took my picture to put in the base newspaper.

The road took me higher and higher, past open spaces and occasional clusters of trees. I saw very few houses until I finally came to a chalet at the top of the mountain. When I learned it would cost $40 to stay overnight, I decided to try to find something less expensive farther up the road. A man who had been watching me as I spoke with the clerk, followed me outside when I left the hotel lobby and tried to talk to me. I heartily wished that I had studied harder in my high school French class or taken the time to learn conversational German. He finally got in his car and left, but stopped out by the road. He was obviously waiting to see which direction I would take.

I felt very uneasy about the him, yet I couldn't just stand there. So I turned right and began pedaling down the road, lined on both sides by dense forests. He passed me and stopped in front of me, opening the car's trunk and indicating that he wanted me to put my bike in. He sounded angry, but might have been simply trying to make me understand him. Without speaking I quietly went around him and kept going. Then I realized that he could stop anywhere up the road again, so I turned around and came back. As I rode past I called to him and pointed to the bike and the sign around my waist, AROUND THE WORLD.

"Oh, oh, oh," he said, appearing surprised.

Since I was still not sure of his intentions, I returned to the hotel. The same girl was at the desk, so I tried to find out if she knew anything about the man. "Yes," she said, but I wondered if she had understood anything I said. After a few minutes I left and started riding. The man was gone, and I never saw him again.

I wondered how I'd know where to stop next. It started to rain, so I left the main road and stopped under the porch of a rather fancy place. It was expensive, but I decided that God knew better than I what I needed. It was important that I soak off the old bandages and apply fresh ones. For that I needed a shower and sanitary conditions in which to work. I needed to wash clothes and get a good night's sleep, too. Safe inside out of the rain and cold, with everything fresh and clean, and my tired body comfortable, I snuggled in for the night, so grateful for that night of restoration.

The next day I left for Karlsruhe. I made good time over the hills and through the valleys, but got off course and ended up too far north. I met a young, English-speaking girl. Claudia invited me to stop and visit in the garden setting on the roof of their business. She also gave me directions to Karlsruhe. I needed to take a ferry across the Rhine River, she said, turn south, and cycle through Blankenburg to Karlsruhe.

Following Claudia's map seemed complicated, but I rolled right along, arriving just in time to catch the small boat that took me across the famous Rhine River. I bent down on the wharf and swished my hand in the water, wondering what stories the ripples would tell if they could only speak. I imagined romance, pleasure boating, and travel along the shore to places offering exotic food and entertainment.

It was getting late when I stopped beside a man on a bicycle at the next intersection. "Which road should I take to find a place to stay tonight?" I asked.

"Why don't you come home with me?" he replied. "My wife and I would be happy to have you."

It took us quite a while to reach his home. He turned here and there in the gathering dusk. Why would I follow a stranger for miles on a bicycle? I can't tell you exactly why, but there was that still, small voice one hears when working side-by-side with the most reliable Travel Agent in the world. When we finally arrived, I realized we'd traveled about five miles to reach Dieter Sanitz's home. His wife, Helga, was just leaving to conduct a fitness class, so he and I enjoyed a simple but satisfying supper of cheese, bread, and several other dishes.

I needed to call Cecilia. Since I didn't understand German or the long-distance phone system, Dieter's help was invaluable. It took several tries to make contact, but he did reach her, and through him I was able to discuss in detail what we should do next. I understood then why God had brought me to his home. Instead of going to Munich and then going south across the

Brenner Pass, I told Cecilia to drive to Basel and we would go over St. Gotthard Pass in the Swiss Alps.

"Everyone here thinks you're crazy for going over that pass, Charlotte," Cecilia said. "The road is so steep over the mountain that bikes use the other route. Because of your commitment to cycle every mile of the way I know you won't ride through the eight-mile tunnel by car, and you know that bicycles are not allowed in there."

I told her I would pray about it and give her an answer very soon. I felt very strongly that I should go through Switzerland and then across the plains of Italy to the Adriatic Sea. My hosts provided me with a lovely upstairs bedroom. I found rest and peace that night, knowing that everything would be all right.

For several days after I left Dieter and Helga, my route followed the Rhine River, past green hillsides and farmlands. Toward evening I stopped at a small market and gas station. I wanted to go to Offenburg Castle in Offenburg. The castle, converted into a youth hostel, had become quite a landmark in the area, but due to the language barrier directions on how to get there proved very confusing. So I stood around and waited to see if someone had a moment to help me. Gabi Blum, who was on her way to English class, offered to take me to the castle. We put my bike in the trunk of her car and set out. The trip took about 30 minutes, with many twists and turns as we went along. One hill was so steep it seemed as if we were going almost straight up. And then we were at the castle, overlooking the city of Offenburg. By now it was dark. I don't think I could have found the place by myself. Plus, I would have had to walk and push my bike to the top.

I secured my bike to the iron railing at the top of the ramp leading into the main castle. My room, which I shared with a young girl, was two stories deep in the earth, reached by winding stairs. The wall had been cut out of solid rock. We shared a bath with two other girls in the room next to ours. These young travelers dressed simply, tying back their long hair, or letting it simply hang loose around their shoulders. Many of them had saved up their money in order to travel to faraway places. I enjoyed hearing them compare notes about places they had visited and about life in general. As they traveled they stayed at hostels, which were much cheaper than hotels. If you have ever hiked, walked, or biked all day long you know how wonderful it felt that night to crawl between fresh sheets, relax, and fall asleep all in one breath.

The next day was Friday, which meant just one more day to go before my day off the road. As I started down the steep hill from the castle I wondered if I'd be able to find my way back to where Gabi had picked me up the day before. I was also concerned about whether or not my brakes would hold on the steep hill. When I finally reached level ground, I let out a deep breath. It took me about an hour to get back to Offenburg. I felt more than a little relieved when I saw the service station where I had stopped the evening before.

Before I left the city I spoke on the telephone with Cecilia again. She had taken care of the van contract through a friend in Munich. The owner had outfitted it with cupboards, a bed, and cooking facilities. It would cost about $800 to rent it, plus gasoline expense.

I filled my water bottles and was soon back on the road, heading south and riding parallel to the fast-moving autobahn. About 5:00 as I cycled into the outskirts of Freiberg, the road simply disappeared. What should I do now? I could see a new road under construction but wasn't sure where it would take me. I stopped at a nearby construction site.

"What can I do for you?" asked the man who came out the door.

When I explained that I needed a place to rest over the next day, he cheerfully suggested that I go home with him, assuring me that his wife and daughter would be happy to have me spend the night. On the way to his home he introduced himself as Gerd E.F.R. Jordan, and mentioned that he and his family planned to go camping the next day. "We belong to a nudist club," he added nonchalantly.

I hid my surprise and asked, "How did you ever get into that?"

"Well, our neighbors belong, and one weekend they invited us to go along. We enjoyed it and have been going ever since."

His wife, Marlene, and daughter, Diane, greeted me warmly. After a lovely supper they showed me to a comfortable guest room where I could spend the night. The next day the family planned to leave about noon to go to the camp. First, however, Marlene took me to the center of Freiberg, where I could visit a famous cathedral in the area. I thanked her again for her family's warm hospitality.

Crowds of people filled the town. The market area offered flowers, vegetables, pastries, and other items for sale. A church choir sang on the small porch of a nearby building. Then someone preached for a while and the choir sang again. Although I couldn't understand a word, I did enjoy the spirit of the event. After I ate lunch and visited with a family from America, I felt I had to get out of the milling throng. The atmosphere wasn't very restful. Although I didn't usually travel on Saturday, it seemed the best way to get out into the country and away from the city. Once there I began to relax, and it didn't take long to put 20 miles between me and the big, bustling city of Freiberg.

Near the town of Bad Krozingen, I saw a couple walking beside a bridge and stopped to ask if they knew of a hostel or guest house in the area. After I explained why I was on the road, they introduced themselves as Mercedes and Siegfried Wille.

Mercedes said, "Why don't you come and stay with us? We live near the river."

The Willes treated me as part of their family. That evening we talked until midnight. When they said they received a religious magazine from America that said the seventh day was the Sabbath, we discussed this and some other religious matters. Mercedes asked me to play some songs on her organ so that she could record them.

I learned that the story of their life was rather unusual. Mercedes had come from South America to visit a married sister in Spain. Siegfried had been a seaman and traveled most of his life. They met through a newspaper notice, fell in love, and married. Their only child, a daughter, planned to visit America to continue her studies in English. We exchanged several letters after I returned to the States, and they have remained a very special part of my memories.

OVER THE TOP

The next morning I was back on Highway 3. I had made my decision: I would climb and ride over the Swiss Alps by way of the

St. Gotthard Pass. When I called Cecilia to tell her of my decision, she reminded me again of the advice she had received against such a crossing. "Charlotte, my friends here say it is very unwise to go that way. Bikes just don't go over the St. Gotthard Pass. It is too hard and too high."

Her discouraging words echoed in my mind as I rode south. I asked people along the way what they thought about the pass. At that point I still had time to turn around and go across to Munich, then south through the Brenner Pass. No one encouraged me to go through St. Gotthard Pass. Their reasons included a little bit of everything: the pass might be closed due to snow, a recent storm had washed out bridges and roads, weather in the pass was very unpredictable.

I realized these people lived in the area and their advice was probably sound. However, I still waited for a definite answer from my unseen Guide. For days I had experienced a strong feeling that I should continue south. Although I should have gone east from Karlsruhe to Munich several days earlier, if that was the best way, a magnet seemed to keep pulling me toward Basel, Switzerland. All voices but One faded into the background. I would climb over the Swiss Alps.

The decision made, I went happily on my way. The ride to the outskirts of Basel was uneventful, and several hours remained until dark when I reached the city. I rode through the traffic, wondering which was the best road to take to the immigration office. When I asked a cheerful-looking gentleman pedaling along beside me for directions, he offered to show me the way. Bless him!

We wove in and out of traffic as I did my best not to lose sight of him in the crowd. When we arrived at the border and customs gate, he rode through without stopping, beckoning for me to follow. Everyone seemed to recognize him and waved us through the gate. When we stopped, I learned that his name was Jerry Gerhasel, chief customs officer for Basel. Jerry stayed with me until we had ridden across town to a hostel located close to the Rhine River. He hooked my bicycle to the railing outside the hostel, then rode away on his own two wheels. Cecilia would join me the next day, driving the van from Munich, and we would meet at the train station. In the meantime, it felt wonderful to be safe inside the hostel.

Most of the next morning was spent writing letters and completing my weekly news bulletin to my son, Gene, who then passed them on to the media and friends. My "office" was a bench beside the Rhine River. As I waited for Cecilia at the station I saw Jerry again. His office was in one area of the immense station. Several hours passed with no sign of Cecilia. Concerned, I called her friend Sonia Navratil in Munich.

"Don't worry," Sonia told me, "she left some time ago, and it is a long way."

Finally, about 8:00 p.m., Cecilia arrived in a yellow van, accompanied by an older gentleman. We didn't know there are two train stations in Basel, and Cecilia had gone to the other station to meet me. The gentleman with her had offered to show her how to get to the right place. We agreed that next time we needed to "read the fine print" before we set out on such an adventure! The important thing was that we were back together and ready to start one of the most exciting adventures of the trip—crossing the Swiss Alps.

We started our journey the next morning under a bright sun shining in a clear, blue sky. How could I help but smile and be cheerful? That afternoon we stopped a little earlier than usual and asked a farmer if we might park in his backyard for the night. He not only agreed, but invited us to eat our supper on a table beneath a small tree in back of the house. Our supper included fresh vegetables from his garden. The hospitable farmer offered us the use of a little bathroom inside the barn. That night I took a bath in a pan of warm water under the gentle scrutiny of nearby cows.

We reached Luzern the next day. Traffic in the busy city was terrible. It was easy to exchange money, though—we even cashed a personal check. Later we stopped at a bar to watch a championship football game between Germany and Denmark. Bars in Europe are general meeting places for everyone, young and old, and not necessarily a place to drink.

Cecilia and I almost became separated again when I stopped for a moment at a public toilet. Just as I returned to the sidewalk I saw her going by in the van. The war whoop I let out caught her attention—and everybody else's for a mile around. A split second later and I would have missed her.

That evening we parked off the road. Despite the clamor of church bells ringing, traffic whizzing by, and trains running all night, we slept surprisingly well. On the road next day I saw the foothills in the distance leading to St. Gotthard Pass. My heart beat a little faster as I realized that if all went well we would reach the summit the next day.

It rained during the night. *It could be snowing up there right now, making it necessary to close the pass,* I thought.

The next afternoon a Swiss soldier stopped Cecilia, who was behind me. "Construction is going on up ahead," he told her. "A severe storm washed out the autobahn and everything else that it could pick up in its path. We've been letting people through this week on makeshift roads, but it is dangerous and difficult. You should go back."

Cecilia didn't budge. "Charlotte Hamlin from the United States is going around the world on a bicycle," she told him. "She's ahead of me—this is her support van. I must stay with her; she needs me."

The soldier allowed her to pass.

I doubt that I will ever forget the scene I saw that afternoon. I had stopped the bike to rest for a moment and looked high above me to the right. A cement ribbon extended across the mad rush of water, then suddenly stopped. The cliffs—and the autobahn—had fallen into the swirling waters below, creating a great chasm. Debris, cement, parts of earth and tree roots made the once-busy freeway look almost like a waterfall as it hung suspended over the edge into space. The bicycle proved to be a blessing in getting around construction vehicles and other obstacles. For me, the adventure was rather exciting. I didn't feel I was in any real danger.

Two German cyclists joined me on the road that day, and we traveled together. We passed through several tunnels built over the road. It was very dark inside, and I realized the danger of hitting a piece of tire or some other object on the side of the road. We passed through in safety, though, and again I offered a silent prayer of thanks. We didn't see Cecilia for quite a while. When she caught up with us she confessed that she'd almost decided to turn around and go back and through the big tunnel.

"My heart surely did some flip-flops on those steep, narrow roads," she told me. "I had to go all the way in first gear and really was afraid that I might not make it."

That evening we pulled into the parking lot of a large Swiss military compound. We decided to park there for the night, wondering if someone would come and chase us away. We invited the German cyclists, Uive Tukemaun and Mike Schweigert, to share a hot meal with us. After supper they rented a room in a nearby bed-and-breakfast establishment and invited us to use the community bathroom in the hallway. A hot soak in the tub and the chance to wash a few clothes were well worth the $3 we paid the landlady.

As I thought about the day that had just passed I realized that the boys showing up gave me some much-needed human support. I felt a twinge of guilt about Cecilia's trip and her anxiety over traveling on the makeshift roads beside the surging river and the heavy equipment. Still, I felt we were on the right track.

Friday morning we heard the sounds of target practice near our overnight parking area. A man informed us that it was illegal for us to park inside the gates of the military compound. The officials were very nice about it, though. I realized I should have looked for the administration building the night before and asked for permission to park overnight.

Cecilia decided to take the 17-kilometer tunnel through the St. Gotthard Pass rather than go over the top as the boys and I planned to do. It was a lovely, sunny day, and we were moving right along about 9:30 when, to my surprise, Cecilia passed us. (She told me later that when she stopped at the tourist office the attendant persuaded her not to miss the thrill of reaching the top and looking out over the world below.)

Uive and I walked most of the distance to the top. Walking was easier than wrestling with the bike all the way. Another gentleman, Klaus, started after we did but caught up with us. We traveled together the rest of the way to the top. I will always be grateful for company on that long, tough climb.

The scenery was absolutely breathtaking. Little Swiss cottages clung to the mountainside. Animals grazed here and there on the steep slopes. There were places where the road we were climbing actually extended into space. Cecilia reached the top ahead of us and without difficulty. When she saw the view, she was glad she had chosen that route. She also enjoyed the opportunity to visit the National Museum with its multimedia presentations. I was sorry there wasn't enough time for me to spend some of the afternoon at the top, but it was important that I reach the foot of the mountain before dark. So I ate a sandwich and rested a bit, then it was time to leave. I was concerned about riding my bike 14½ miles down the other side of the mountain. Uive had ridden my bike a short distance going up and told me the brakes were not very good. I remembered that the repairman at the bike shop in Belgium wasn't sure he had repaired the brakes properly. This was not the best place to have his doubts confirmed.

When someone mentioned my concern about the brakes, Klaus said he had the special tool needed to fix them. It took him about an hour to complete the job. What if he hadn't brought the tool with him that day? What if he hadn't chosen that day to climb the mountain? God had sent me yet another blessing!

The others were eager to be on their way as they had plans for the evening. I assured them I would be all right, and they soon disappeared around the bend in the road and were soon out of sight. I left about 2:00 p.m. Cecilia would meet me later. At first I braked constantly to make sure that I stayed in control and was going slowly enough to make it around the constant series of corners as the road curved back and forth all the way to the bottom. I had to pump the brakes so they wouldn't overheat. Constant caution was my watchword. A low, two-foot guardrail was on one side of the road, a high cliff on the other. Once I started to look around a little at the scenery, then remembered my accident in Luxembourg and reminded myself to look straight ahead. If I were to hit something in the road there was nothing to stop me from being catapulted from the seat of the cycle to the valley 1,000 feet below.

The trip down took little time compared to the trip up the mountain. A road made of cobblestones at the bottom provided some rough going for a while, and I wondered if I would make Biasca before sunset. Cecilia found me at the post office in Pollegio about 5:30. It was getting late, so I put the bike on the van and we decided to spend the night at Al Censo Campground. I'd been praying for a place that had a long-distance phone and English-speaking people. I needed to call Gene and notify him of our progress. God answered my prayer. The campground managers, Peter and Magrit Grentert, spent part of each year in America and spoke very good English. I gave Gene our exciting progress report and, just as important, learned that all was well at home.

The next day was my day to rest. The rain that started Friday night continued all day Saturday and into Sunday morning. Sunday, September 27, was my 69th birthday, although I didn't feel any different than I had for the past 50 years. *Who knows? I* thought. *If I take care of myself there might be 30 more years of good health.* It was great to be doing what I wanted to do, being what I wanted to be, and going where I wanted to go. Health is a wonderful gift, something worth reaching out for and cherishing.

We did a little housecleaning after breakfast, bought a few items, and were ready to be on our way. We planned to cross the border into Italy that day.

ITALY AND THE ADRIATIC

We arrived in Italy on Sunday evening and parked on the outskirts of Chiasso, a town not far from the border. So much had happened in the past few days. I knew that the Swiss Alps would remain in my memory as a friend, not a foe. The day after we went through St. Gotthard's Pass it was closed because of snow. Cecilia and I discovered anew it pays to trust God, no matter how many voices are singing a different song. We planned to drive through Brenner Pass on the way home to return the yellow camper to its owner in Munich. That way, we'd have the opportunity to see both worlds.

On the 60 miles from Chiasso to Bergamo I enjoyed a restful trip biking beside Lake Lugano. I waited for Cecilia at Fort Loll, but no yellow camper appeared. Someone said they thought she had passed that way about an hour earlier. With the heavy traffic and so many people it seemed impossible not to become lost. Our paths finally crossed about 4:30, then Cecilia left to buy groceries.

I reached Bergamo about dusk. Roads spoked out in every direction from the hub of the city. When you can't read the signs, tell how much money is in your hand, or get an answer that means anything, what do you do next? I ended up at the train station in Treviglio and went into a nearby pizza parlor to ask if anyone had seen the yellow camper. No one had, so I sat down at the counter and ordered a pizza. Tired and cold, I wondered what to do next. Finally, I decided to go back to the train station. A policeman, De Roberto Antonio, offered to stay with me while I waited for the van.

Cecilia had contacted the police when she first arrived in Bergamo. "There was a maze of roads out there—not even a rat would know how to find its way!" she declared. "And I always had that fear that someone could have kidnapped you or hit you—all kinds of dreadful things were dancing through my head."

Mario Bononie, a young man who spoke English, took her to his restaurant to wait. Eventually, a call from the police came through and the restaurant owner brought Cecilia to the train station, where she found me surrounded by a group of young people. We all returned to Mario's restaurant and enjoyed a visit with him over a dish of fresh grapefruit. Young people filled the restaurant. Mario remarked that "parents here give their young people a lot of money, but they have nothing to do."

Our host called a policeman friend and asked if he would let us park in his courtyard for the night. Cecilia felt uneasy about the arrangement, but we were in a large city, it was getting late, and it seemed OK to me. His place was quite far away, and Cecilia's concern increased as we followed him through narrow streets, around obstacles, and then into an extremely narrow alley with high walls on both sides. In the dim light the policeman got out and opened a thick wooden door. After we drove through, the door creaked shut behind us and was secured by a heavy bar.

The cracked cement walls of the courtyard were crumbling in some places. On one side it looked as if small openings for windows had been left in the thick walls. A stairway led to the upper level. Cecilia said she felt like a captive in that dark place, but it was late and we finally crawled into bed.

All was well the next morning, although Cecilia still felt uneasy until we were on the other side of that heavy swinging door. There is really no good place to hide from danger. People can help us find security behind high walls, but trusting God in all circumstances removes a lot of everyday stress that constantly confronts us. We can always rest in the assurance that we have nothing to fear as long as we are doing His will.

I returned to the train station so that I could resume my journey from where I had stopped the night before. As I traveled to Cremona I couldn't help noticing the difference from the green hills and hamlets of Switzerland. Restroom accommodations were poor, often having no toilet paper or soap, and sometimes no water. Debris littered the highways, and buildings needed repairs. We learned later that people in the north of Italy were poorer than those in the south. The people, however, were always friendly and helpful.

Cecilia came along about midmorning. We were both enjoying the warmer weather. Our spirits lifted as we left the high mountains behind and crossed the plains on our way to the sea and a new adventure.

At 4:00 Cecilia and her yellow van met me outside Cremona. She had a couple policemen with her. *Vittoreano Zanolli,* a newspaper in Cremona, sent someone to interview me. We were also allowed to park there overnight. In Italy it seemed to be the in thing to pull up anywhere there was a place to park and stay for the night.

Cecilia moaned, "This middle-aged, German-born American wishes she could speak some Italian!" That day she had passed a museum that housed 44 Stradivarius violins. She had wanted to stop and see them, but the fee to get in was quite high.

It was September 30. Fall had arrived, and we needed to hurry and finish our trip before it got too cold. The road across the plains from Cremona to Ostiglia was very flat. As I rode I noticed that walls surrounded most dwellings and bars covered the windows. Cecilia caught up with me at noon at an outdoor market. We enjoyed a stew made of vegetables and garbanzo beans, a good source of protein and roughage. Cecilia passed me at 5:00 p.m., then waited for me at the Esso station. The station manager put my bike inside for the night.

I wanted a loaf of real whole-wheat bread, and we finally found a bakery. When they didn't have the real thing we settled for some doughy rolls and long, twisted apple cakes. At least we had bread and water! We turned in at 8:00, laughing and joking over nothing.

The next day we were in wine country. Vineyards covered much of the land, although orchards dominated some areas. We stopped at a farm in Ravenna that night.

The Adriatic Sea area provided some variety in the scenery. Riding past freshly plowed fields or across rolling hills in the cool fall air with the bright sun above brought an inner feeling of peace and gratitude for the new experiences of each day. Cecilia went on ahead to San Marino, where she planned to mail some letters from the small independent state. I was to follow along the beach beside the sea, and she was to find me there after she left San Marino. We should have checked out the small coastal highway before we separated. The winding side roads were dead-end in some places, and simply ceased to exist in others. There was nothing for me to do but follow the main road. I wondered how Cecilia would ever find me. I finally reached Pesaro, a fairly large town near the waterfront. I waited a while, then decided to check into a hotel, where I enjoyed a hot bath and slept in a nice warm bed. There was only one problem: where was my driver?

She was about 60 miles south of Pesaro, in Senigallia. Two men took her to the police station, but it wasn't open. She talked to the Senigallia talk box (outside phone) and waited there for further information. When the men had to leave, Cecilia stood alone in the darkness of a dead-end alley. She spotted a fenced-in, gloomy-looking police station and went inside. A teenager served as an interpreter while she explained her problem to the officers. They

About 1930.
Here we all are!
Arthur, Charlotte (me),
George, and the twins,
Marion and Ruth—
or is it Ruth and Marion?

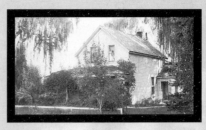

This is our family home in
Canada, where I grew up.

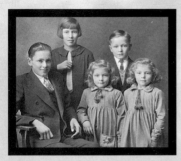

I had written
"middle-aged" on
the back of this picture.
But I've crossed that out
and written "still young."

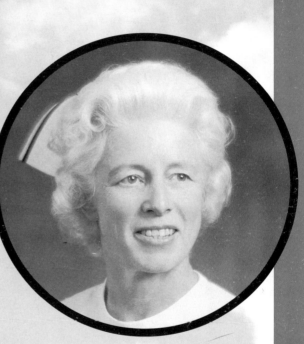

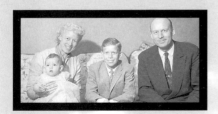

1954-1960: We were missionaries
in Japan. I'm holding Ladonna.
Beside me are Gene Jr. and Gene Sr.

Springtime
1946. My
husband,
Gene, and I.

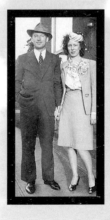

RWTW-4

F A M I L Y

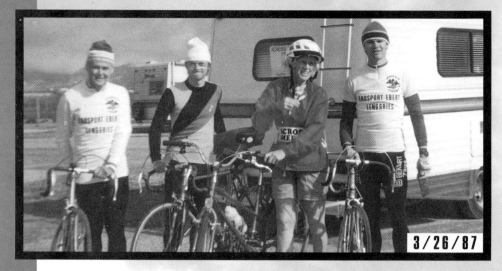

3/26/87

The Van Horns (father and sons) from Germany
were spending their vacation cycling across the U.S.

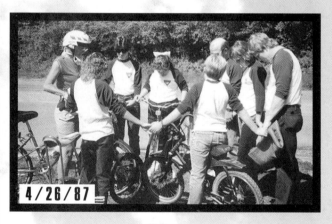

4/26/87

The Roebuck
Pathfinder Club
praying for my safety
(near Birmingham,
Alabama).

I stopped for lunch at Piedmont
Park near Atlanta, Georgia.

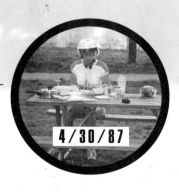

4/30/87

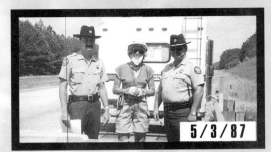

With my good friends, the Georgia state troopers. They told me I was "illegal" (for riding on the interstate) but since I was only five miles from the border they let me go with a "ride safely!" (Note my "smog" mask.)

5/3/87

The finish line: Folly Beach, Charleston, South Carolina. I shall always cherish this picture. Two gulls share my joy in having finished a task I set out to accomplish.

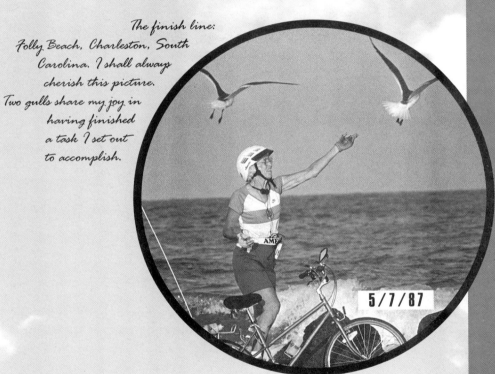

5/7/87

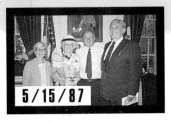

5/15/87

On the way home I met New York City's Mayor Koch. He asked if he could come with me across Europe. I said, "Of course!"

I'm ready to start my trip through Europe. Nieuwpoort, Belgium's, director of tourism presented pewter plates to my driver, Cecilia Seabury, and me. The plates are imprinted with the city's seal.

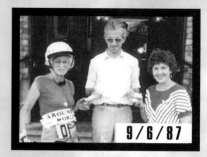

9/6/87

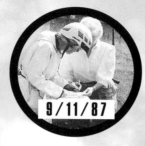

9/11/87

People would sometimes stop me on the road and ask for my autograph!

Sandweiler, Luxembourg. I was watching for a road sign and hit the curb, badly scraping my right arm and upper thigh. Danielle and Claude Branco-Weber offered me assistance and cleaned and bandaged my wounds. Preve Schlmitt, the city's mayor, took this picture of us.

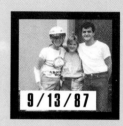

9/13/87

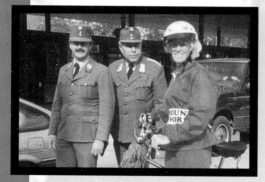

Swiss authorities at the border crossing.

Finish point, Otranto, Italy. The Basilica Cathedral, built around 1080, bears an inscription stating that St. Peter once evangelized Otranto.

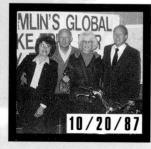

10/20/87

Home again! Cecilia and I were met at Chicago's O'Hare airport by Gene Sr. and Gene Jr.

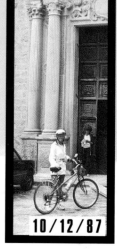

10/12/87

Leaving for Asia. Tracing the route I'll take through Israel, India, and Nepal.

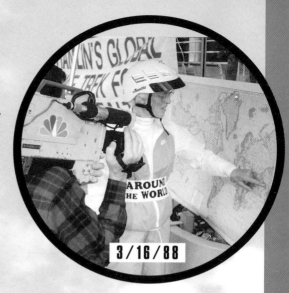

3/16/88

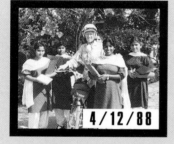

4/12/88

I spoke to 400 students at the Pakistan Adventist Seminary. Later, as I rode away, the students showered me with rose petals.

Katmandu, Nepal. Paul, Dawn, Joel, and Michelle Dulhunty. This family has changed the lives of 2,000 lepers here. Paul is the Nepal ADRA director.

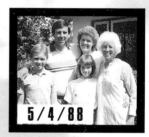

5/4/88

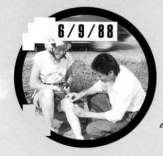

6/9/88

As Wong Gong and I were returning from a visit to China's Great Wall, our bikes collided and I got another deep gouge in my poor left knee.

China's interior. The diet of these wonderfully healthy, hardworking people is mostly vegetables, some fruit, bread, and meat as a seasoning.

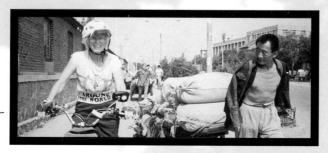

Southeast China. One of the few accidents I saw in China. The driver of this truck fell asleep at the wheel.

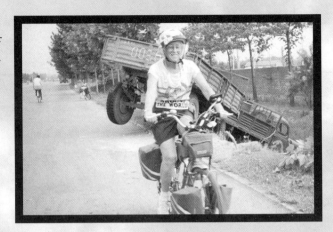

China's interior. Crossing the Yellow River. Very little traffic here.

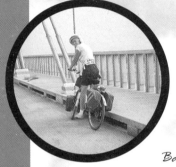

On the road from Bangkok to Singapore. Billboards have even found their way out here!

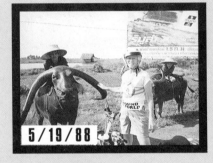

5/19/88

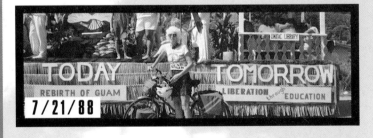

TODAY
REBIRTH OF GUAM

TOMORROW
LIBERATION through EDUCATION

7/21/88

I got to Guam in time to join their parade!

Sydney, Australia. Finishing point of my Australian trip. The Sydney Opera House is behind me.

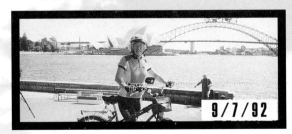

9/7/92

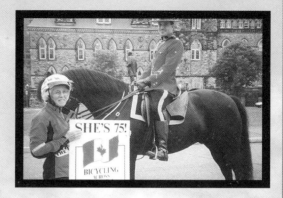

The sign says it all!

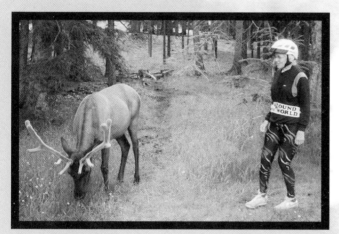

I think I could almost pet him . . .

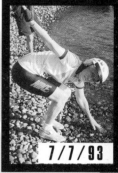

7/7/93

I dip my hand in the Pacific Ocean to officially begin my Canada tour!

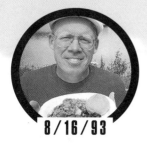

8/16/93

"Chef" Gene displays some of his cooking during a lunch break near Keewatin, Ontario.

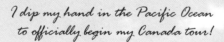

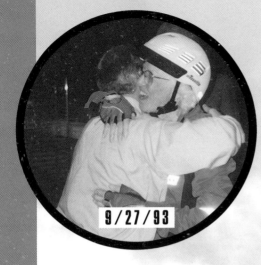

9/27/93

My 75th birthday.
I get a big hug from
the mayor of Charlottetown,
Prince Edward Island.
Nice name for a town!

Carl Baudreau and
his mechanic fixed
up my bike after it
had been vandalized.

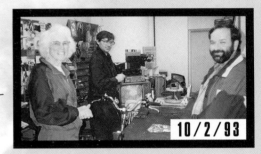

10/2/93

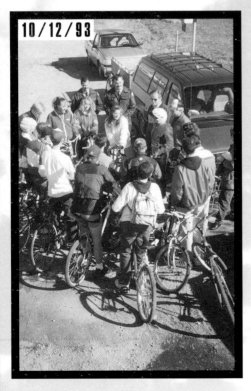

10/12/93

End of the Canadian
journey! Two officers from
the Royal Newfoundland
Constabulary brief me and
students and teachers from
St. John's Academy on the
eight-mile route we'll be
taking to City Hall.

Senior citizens
can do more
than rock!
They can
roll—across
4,200 miles in
10 provinces.

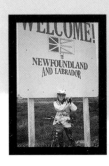

contacted law enforcement agencies and hospitals from Rimini to Ancona, looking for me. The police suggested she go back to Pesaro, but she decided to stay in Senigallia and sleep in the camper.

The next day was our rest day. I went to the police station on the flower-filled main city square. I was interested in only one thing: finding Cecilia. The police located her in Senigallia. When she arrived at the police station in Pesaro, I introduced her to the officers and a young female interpreter who had been a great help. We thanked them and left, knowing we had to find a way to keep from becoming separated again. Cecilia really ribbed me about going off to a nice warm hotel and leaving her out in the cold camper. In my defense I pointed out that I'd have had to really fly low to make it all the way to Senigallia. We had fun blaming each other.

We went down to the beach and walked along the shore where we visited with a wedding party. We soaked in the sounds of the waves gently lapping against the sand and the crying seagulls soaring overhead. The time spent there helped both of us to relax. We picked up the bike and were walking back to the camper when Cecilia started to experience a lot of pain in her right hip. I tried to give her a ride on the carrier of the bike, but that didn't turn out too well. We were in heavy traffic, and the bike wiggled so much that I was afraid she would end up with more than a sore hip. It was a relief when we finally reached the camper. We parked on the wharf for the night. The Algida bar/snack shop across from us allowed me to leave my cycle in their shop overnight. Groups of people walked by on the promenade late into the night.

Sunday's travel took us through little villages snuggled in the coves and near the beaches all along the Adriatic. Cecilia passed me around noon, and we had lunch near Ancona. I had covered nearly 40 miles by 1:00 p.m. We stopped that night at a bar/cafe. We bought a few things to eat, but healthy food is hard to come by in most parts of the world, especially if one is just going down the road and wants to find something in a hurry.

The next day's travel took us on a winding road through dense green forests. At one point two cars stopped in the middle of the road and the drivers came over to get a closer look at this white-haired senior citizen. Cars began to pile up behind them, causing quite a traffic jam.

It was getting harder to find a place to bathe, wash clothes, and generally meet our needs. We considered taking a side trip by boat to Greece, about a 24-hour ride. There really wasn't much time left, however, and we also had to consider the cost. We decided to forgo the trip to Greece.

We'd been back on the road for some time when I began to wonder whether Cecilia was ahead of me or behind. Sometimes she stopped to do a little sightseeing or shopping. From past experience I knew how easy it was for me to go by and not notice the yellow van. When I saw a police car parked beside the road, I asked the officer if he'd seen her. He radioed headquarters and, sure enough, she was there. This was the first time she had gone to a police station in the daytime. With two officers leading the way, we hurried down the street, across corners, and through intersections, switching lanes constantly. I broke every sensible rule of biking trying to keep up with them in the heavy traffic. We arrived at the police station safely, and once again Cecilia and I were together.

Cecilia had met a family on the outskirts of town who impressed her as being special, and she wanted me to meet them. Their cafe, a tent with bamboo sides, was open from April to November. Then they closed the cafe and went to the mountains to ski for four months.

For supper they served us vegetables. The green peppers had been peeled and oiled, then broiled on a very hot grill. I hoped the family didn't live on this fare regularly since benzoapyrene is a carcinogen and many times more concentrated than the same poison found in cigarettes. However, I don't consider it my assignment to line up someone else's life for them. Each one of us is responsible for the choices we make. I do know that drugs such as alcohol, tobacco, and coffee, although acceptable in our society, can cause arrhythmia of the heart, bladder cancer, possibly breast cancer, and many other illnesses. My motto is simple: if it damages, don't do it.

The next morning I learned a valuable lesson: don't ever fasten your bicycle to the doorknob of a van. That's what I had done before going to bed—and we started off the next morning with the bike still fastened to the door. It seemed to take forever to come to a stop and get around to view the damage. The front wheel was bent a little, so we stopped at a bicycle shop that was right down the road. We decided to go to a bank to cash some travelers checks while they worked on the bike. A very nice lady offered to drive ahead of us to show us the way. One of the employees spoke English and helped us handle our business, then wished us well on our trip.

With the bike repaired, we were back on the road again. The police were stopping traffic at one point—I wasn't sure why they stopped everyone—but when I showed them some pictures and an article about me written in German they allowed me to continue on my way. When Cecilia came by later, they also questioned her very closely.

One very sad thing I noticed on the road was the markers showing the places where accidents had taken lives, mostly of young men. Sometimes flowers lay beside their pictures or a spiritual thought in a little enclosed space. And sometimes there was a bottle of wine or other drink. I don't remember seeing any markers placed out there for girls, although there must have been some.

We stopped overnight at a home in the country. Three generations lived in that house that had withstood the wind and weather for many a century. The family helped me telephone home and wish my daughter, Ladonna, a happy birthday. It was October 8, and we had only a few days left before we would reach the end of our journey.

For mile after mile the next day big trucks loaded with grapes passed me. I bought a few grapes at a roadside stand. Delicious! By the time it got dark I was ready to leave the road. It was dangerous to be out there in the dark, and I already had many hours and miles behind me for the day. Just outside Bari I stopped by a well-drilling business on the other side of a storm fence. Using my best shouting voice I asked if they'd seen a yellow camper from Germany pass by. They hadn't, but the owner's son overheard me asking. On his way home, he went to a gas station about three miles down the road. Sure enough, Cecilia was there. What timing!

She came back with the young man, and the manager allowed us to park inside their fenced-in area for the night and put my bike inside the building. I was a bit cautious around their two watchdogs at first—I didn't want to finish the trip with one leg. We talked nicely to them and fed them a few bites of food.

The next morning I reached for my water bottle to fill it up before beginning the day's travel. It was gone! I checked up and down the road and finally found it, minus its cap, bent from being run over by traffic. It had served me well. I would save it, along with my worn-out sweater, shoes, and other mementoes.

About midafternoon outside Brindisi we put the bike on the rack and decided to take some time to catch up on other things that needed our attention. We were already in the heel of Italy's "boot" and would cross the finish line by Monday morning if all went well. We parked next to the harbor and looked out over the sea. Greece was on the other side of that expanse of water. Would I return here someday to ride east with the wind at my back, not stopping until I had gone full circle around the globe?

We walked down the street, past open-air cafes filled with noisy throngs of tourists and milling townspeople. In a small cafe we had lunch with Dorothy, a 63-year-old retired professor from south of Darmstadt. She and her Dalmatian were traveling by themselves in a huge Mercedes camper. Her husband was currently on another trek somewhere else, she said, and she planned to spend three or four weeks in Greece, researching into the arts and archaeology of the country.

Later that day Cecilia and I went down to watch the boat leave for Greece and tell Dorothy goodbye. I noticed a large group of young people going aboard on the lower deck, carrying backpacks filled with sleeping bags, food, and other equipment. I guessed they were out to see the world before home duties hemmed them in.

The next day a journalist from the *Gazzetta De Mezzogioruo* came to interview me for the paper. In the afternoon we walked on the beach, enjoying the warm fall sunshine. That evening we watched Francesco Moser in a cyclist race in Moscow on a television set in the harbor pilot's office.

The next morning Cecilia and I read about Paul in the New Testament. His sea experiences while en route to Rome were just one miracle after another. What a godly man! Nothing could destroy him until his work was done. On a steep hillside out the window to our left stood a huge monument that marked the end of the Appian Way. The other terminal of this famous road was in Rome. This sight was not a memory that time would erase, but one to renew in our hearts the story of the man taken outside Rome on the other end of this same trail and beheaded for being a follower of Christ. Paul knew he was on his way to die, but declared, "I have fought the good fight, I have finished the race, I have kept the faith. Now there is in store for me the crown of righteousness, which the Lord, the righteous Judge, will award to me on that day—and not only to me, but also to all who have longed for his appearing" (2 Timothy 4:7, 8, NIV).

This would be our last full day on the road. I was heading east toward our final destination. As I cycled along the road I found myself thinking back over the trip. What could I have done differently? Did the peace I had found through faith in God encourage anyone along the way to trust in Him too? Was my simple lifestyle a positive example in helping others accept what they could not change?

Along the route a number of small fortresses stood vacant and in disrepair. Refuse bordered each side of the road, and flies swarmed everywhere. While traveling along a clean, well-landscaped freeway was certainly more uplifting to the spirits, here I didn't have as many speeding semis or as much smog.

Cecilia and I arrived at the gateway of Missionari Comboniani at the same time. A light mist fell from the overcast sky, the wind blew, and the whole outdoors felt cold and clammy. We had no idea what type of mission it was. Should we go inside? I knocked on the door. The priest who answered the door invited us to enter, explaining it was a training center for youth who would go to North Africa to work. Two of the priests, P. Gianni Stirparo and Ciccarese Stirparo, were brothers. They served us a soft drink and some biscuits while we rested. Several nuns and students came by to meet us and visit. One of the women took us to a room in another part of the building, where we were welcome to stay for the night. Until you've lived in a camper with the nights getting colder and the space inside seeming to get smaller, you can't appreciate how wonderful it feels to be inside, curled up in a warm bed, all clean and happy.

Monday, October 12. The big day had arrived! The gentle rain kept me cool as I gave the last day everything I had. A silent prayer of thanks rose from my heart. *Thank You for good weather most of the time, and for protection from serious injury and other dangers through 1,800 miles of wheel turning between the coast of Belgium and the bottom of the boot.*

In Brindisi someone suggested that I finish at the Otranto Cathedral located at the top of a very steep hill in Otranto. It took just over two hours to go the 25 miles, including pushing my bike to the top of the small mountain. At the top of the mountain Cecilia started to drive through a narrow tunnel to get to the courtyard. The tunnel was so narrow that she panicked and stopped right in the tunnel. Cars began to back up behind her. Finally two young men rescued her, one driving the van, while the other gave directions. She was almost in shock by the time she reached me.

Otranto is the farthest eastward point of Italy, open to every invasion, and unprotected from any attack from the sea. In 1480 the inhabitants, firm in the love of their faith and fatherland, refused the proposals of the Turkish Fleet of Mohammed. Twenty thousand people were slaughtered on the walls, along the streets, and in the cathedral itself. Eight hundred survivors had to choose between denying Christ or being beheaded. They chose death. Their remains lie buried in the Chapel of the Martyrs, along with the wooden block on which they were beheaded.

The front part of the church has stood since the fifteenth century, and the doorway entrance since 1674. As I stepped on the mosaic pavement at the front entrance I realized I stood on an authentic masterpiece. Eleven hundred years before, a Greek artist had portrayed the stories of the Bible in the mosaics, from the time of Adam and Eve in the Garden. A large, rectangular hole in the far corner of the next room was a baptismal font from about 300 A.D.

The inscription stated that Saint Peter, the prince of the apostles, had once evangelized Otranto.

Across the square Cecilia and I met the mayor and other city officials. The mayor's photographer took pictures, and his wife accompanied us to the shores of the Adriatic Sea down in the village. I took off my shoes and socks and waded out into the sea. A feeling of relief came over me as I realized that it was all over. At the same time my gaze traveled across the water to another part of the world not too far away.

The next morning we began the trip home, traveling north along the coast, then across the mountains through Brenner Pass. Though not as steep as St. Gotthard Pass, our present route was more up- and downhill. As we traveled across Austria's emerald mountainsides, dotted with alpine homes, my heart filled with gratitude for the gift of life. At the border between Austria and Germany the press interviewed me for a newspaper story. I had my picture taken with the Austrian inspectors dressed in all their finery, but the Germans didn't want to have their pictures taken in uniform.

In Munich Cecilia's old friends, the Navratils, welcomed us into their home. We cleaned the camper and returned it to the owners. Our timing in returning to Luxembourg was nothing short of a miracle. Horst Navratil had several days off work, giving him time to take us to Luxembourg, as well as enjoying a little relaxation and fun with his family on the way home.

The two Genes (my husband and my son) met us at O'Hare International Airport in Chicago, and soon we were back home in Berrien Springs, Michigan. Soon I was "back in the harness," conducting health education classes.

Would the way open up to continue my dream to ride with the wind, always facing the sunrise, until I once again reached the Pacific shoreline where it had all begun?

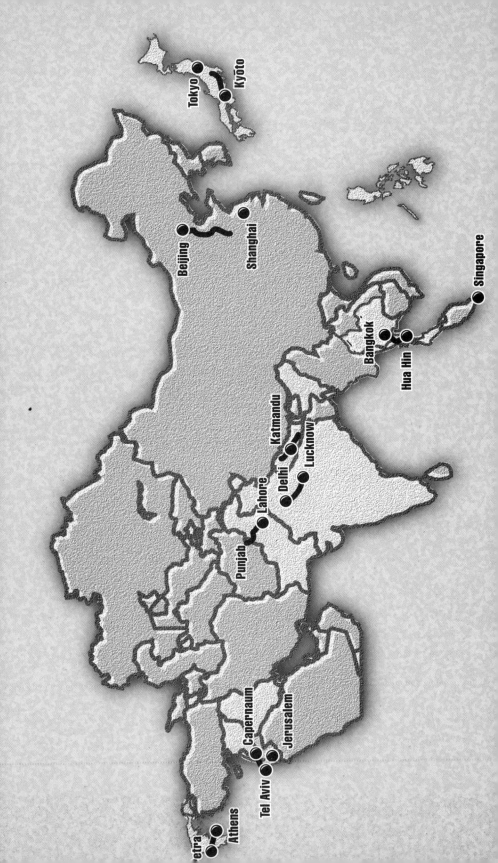

THROUGH PARTS OF ASIA *March 16–September 27, 1988*

Tokyo
Kyōto
Beijing
Shanghai
Singapore
Bangkok
Hua Hin
Katmandu
Lucknow
Delhi
Lahore
Punjab
Capernaum
Jerusalem
Tel Aviv
Athens
Petra

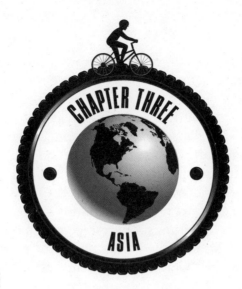

CHAPTER THREE

ASIA

ON THE WAY, ALONE

January 1988 brought typical Michigan cold and snow. Everyone else in the family was busy with his or her own interests, so I decided it was a good time to finish my dream.

I planned to leave for Athens, Greece, the middle of March. I would then travel through parts of Greece, the Holy Land, Pakistan, India, Nepal, Thailand; China, Japan, Guam, and Hawaii. I thought that if I went to Washington, D.C., and got all my visas at one time the rest would be easy. I needed $300 to cover my airfare and lodging, but didn't have that much cash available at the time. Just before I was to leave I received a partial refund of my Medicare health premium. The amount? Three hundred dollars!

In Washington everything fell into place for me. I shared a taxi from the airport with another lady who insisted on paying my fare, then tucked a gift of $20 into my hand. The Mennonite hostel where I stayed was delightful. They served fresh muffins, cereal, and orange juice for breakfast, as well as refreshments in the evening after vespers. Their work is a real service of love.

Within the week I had visas for several countries and information on how to get the other visas I needed. Back in Berrien Springs speaking engagements at the Kiwanis Club, the United Methodist Women's Club, the Women's Reading Guild, and other groups kept me busy. I didn't charge for these appearances, but if someone gave me an honorarium it went into our nonprofit organization.

My son, Gene, helped me assemble a packet for my itinerary. We sent one to Victor Cooper at the Seventh-day Adventist head- quarters in Washington, D.C., who was in charge of public relations for the world field. His secretary then sent information to church offices in different parts of the world about the time of my arrival.

On my retirement income, I knew I couldn't afford to spend four or five months in Asia. I prayed that God would supply the means for me to go if my trip would honor His name. We did send out a few letters requesting sponsorship, which Gene followed up with phone calls. Meanwhile, I went right on with my preparations as though the money were already in my pocket. At the medical center I received shots for typhoid, cholera, tetanus, and gamma globulin. I was also given a blood test and pills to prevent malaria.

Preparation for the trip included extensive planning, as I would be alone most of the time in Asia. Everything must be as light as possible, as I must carry everything needed for daily travel on the bicycle. I would have to carry my cooking utensils, summer and winter clothes, extra shoes, rain jacket, an extra tire and tube, small tools, an extra cable, and a small towel. The bicycle shop or- dered four panniers that fitted on carriers on the bike frame. Flat on one side and rounded on the other, the streamlined panniers offered less wind resistance.

I realized that people in some of the countries I would be rid- ing through had never seen a touring, 15-speed Schwinn Mirada. I would need God's protection along the way so that nothing would happen to the frame or other parts that could not be replaced. We ordered a waist banner that I would wear like a wide belt with the words AROUND THE WORLD printed on both the front and back. Students and professors from Andrews University's cos- mopolitan community, representing more than 80 countries, helped me make out a sheet listing in several languages the words and phrases I would need to use.

My flight schedule ran several pages long. We had to confirm reservations with a number of different airlines along the way. When the newspaper ran an article stating that I would leave the next week, I still needed $4,000 for the airline tickets. Nevertheless, we continued to operate on faith that everything would fall into place.

On March 8 Gene Jr. and I had an appointment to see Steve Upton, public relations director at Whirlpool Corporation in Benton Harbor, Michigan. Through the years the Upton family, well-known in the area, had unselfishly given of their means to help in both large and small projects. The next day a check for $5,000 arrived as a donation from the family. About the same time a check for $4,000 arrived from Ellsworth McKee, president of McKee Baking Company in Tennessee. These two gifts, along with several smaller donations, provided enough for my ticket, some travel money, and for Gene's expenses in connection with notifying the media and others he needed to keep informed by writing bulletins.

Traveler's checks amounting to $2,400 would take care of me for five months out on the road. I planned to stay in hostels and primitive inns. Sometimes people would invite me to their homes, and sometimes I would spend the night on a compound where missionaries served. Other times national workers or native people in the lands where I traveled would take me in as one of the family. Many times only God could have directed me where I should go. I ate simple foods and didn't buy "things." In this way, I would return home with $50 left. It's hard to tell how these things happen, but there is one thing about which I'm sure: as long as I return to God one-tenth of my own earnings (which are really His anyway), He makes sure that the remainder takes care of my needs.

Before I left I wanted to make a quick trip to Ohio to visit my granddaughter and Steve, my son-in-law. My daughter, Ladonna, was in school in Seattle; we had said our goodbyes earlier. The delay would disrupt my schedule in some places, but I felt I needed the extra few days to finish preparations and say goodbye.

On departure day we held a press conference at the Marriott Hotel, covered by Channels 16 and 22. I showed a short movie that had been made in Atlanta about my trip across America, and renewed my commitment to promote health and healing along the way as I traveled. When Gene took me to lunch afterward he seemed very solemn and sad. Cecilia and her son, Bruce, came down to help us get everything off to a good start. The two men put my bike in a box. We organized and checked the baggage. After several rounds of hugs, kisses, and goodbyes I boarded the plane. For a moment a small edge of doubt washed over me. I felt very alone and wondered if it was right to put Gene through this ordeal. He knew I'd been cautioned about bandits in China, thieves in India, and unrest in the Punjab in Pakistan. How could I possibly make it alone? I found out later that big man that he is, Gene broke down and cried on Cecilia's shoulder as the plane lifted off. "I don't think that I'll ever see her again," he told her.

After the long flight across the Atlantic I spent two nights at Enton Hall, a live-in center on a mountainside near London. It was fun seeing how these places were run, and it also helped me orient myself for the big task ahead of me. I managed a quick trip into London to see the changing of the guard and to attend vespers at Westminster Abbey.

Security seemed especially heavy when I left the Gatwick airport on Sunday. I hoped the baggage people would take my bike the way it was without loosening the pedals or handlebars and possibly stripping the threads. Happily, they asked me only to take off one pedal and to let some of the air out of the tires. (Air pressure in the baggage compartment could cause a tire to explode.)

En route to Frankfurt, a lady seated across the aisle gave some of my pictures to the chief stewardess who then took them to the captain. He moved me to first class! The stewardess took my résumé to include in the TWA newsletter that goes wherever TWA flies. What a way to tell the world about health!

Norbert Doratek from the Seventh-day Adventist conference office in Frankfurt met me at the airport. What a relief to have someone help me get the bike from the airport to my quarters! I planned to stop in Frankfurt long enough for interviews at a radio station, newspaper, and a magazine. Norbert took me to dinner at the Seventh-day Adventist Christian school in Darmstadt. Afterward, we visited the apartment where Yvonne, my Frankfurt hostess, lived. She worked at the conference office also.

The time came for my interviews. After putting air in the bike's tires and replacing the pedal, I loaded my panniers and got my helmet. I put on my beautiful yellow-and-white bike suit (a gift from Niki) with lots of white zippers and started out in a drizzling rain to ride the short distance to the Voice of Hope radio station, my first appointment of the afternoon. The props were all in place when I arrived. Bert Hensel from the *Darmstadter Echo* needed a picture to accompany his article. I had on my AROUND THE WORLD banner and other gear. Bert took pictures as I rode up and down the road, stood by the bike, or blew the whistle that I carried around my neck for emergencies. Prior to my arrival another story had been written about my stopover in Germany and my plans for the next four months. These pictures would go along with the news story.

By 2:30 we were in the studio, and Elizabeth Neufeld, a Russian journalist, interviewed me for the Voice of Hope. The interview would be beamed through Italy and Portugal to Russia, as well as translated into German and aired throughout Germany. I hoped my life could be an example to youth who so often live only for today, and for all who are too busy to take care of their precious, irreplaceable health.

THE ANCIENT LAND OF GREECE

Before I left the next morning I discarded some items I didn't want and sent home others I didn't need. (If only I'd followed my own advice in the first place I wouldn't be whittling down already!) A young man from the conference office drove me to the airport and helped me get settled on the plane. Everyone had been so organized and caring—I felt like part of the family. My seatmate, a Pan Am engineer, told me he had assisted with the space shuttle *Columbia* that exploded before it reached orbit. He was there, saw the explosion at the site, and watched as the debris floated back to earth. An unforgettable experience.

En route to Athens we flew over the snow-covered Austrian Alps—breathtakingly beautiful. Later we flew over the spot in the white-blanketed countryside below us where Italy, Austria, and Switzerland come together.

When the customs officer in Athens saw me with my bike and panniers, he waved me through without opening my gear. No one was there to meet me, so I called the conference office and learned that because of the heavy smog in the city people were being required to take turns driving their cars. Those with even-numbered license plate numbers drove on even-numbered days; owners of odd-numbered license plates drove on odd-numbered days. The office had an even license number—and this was March 23. So I put my possessions on the bike racks and launched out into the traffic, praying that everything would fall into place. A short distance from the airport I stopped two young girls to ask about a hotel for the night. They introduced themselves as Julie and Claire from London and said they had come to Athens to work in the pubs where U.S. servicemen congregated in the evenings.

"There's a hotel in the direction you just came from," said Julie.

"I don't like to travel in the opposite direction from where I'm going if I can help it," I told them. "You don't suppose there's something up this way?"

"Why don't you come home with us?" Claire offered.

We walked back to the apartment they shared with two other girls. The place was small and things were a little hectic, but I appreciated their hospitality. That night they took me to the pub where they worked. On the way home we stopped to see two of their friends, Carol and Forrest. Carol also worked in the pub, and Forrest was a bomb demolition expert. Although Carol and Forrest invited me to stay with them in their guest room, I wanted to show my appreciation to the other girls and declined their offer. Julie insisted I take her bed, and she slept with one of her roommates.

The next morning Carol came over in her car, even though it was not her day to be on the streets. She said Forrest insisted she take me out to the road that I must take to get to Petra. So I put my bike in the trunk of the car and we rode to the outskirts of the city, past the Parthenon and other famous landmarks. I realized

Carol was taking a chance of being fined for driving on the wrong day, just to help me. What a girl!

After she left, an empty feeling came over me as I stood near the side of the road. I checked the pressure in the bicycle tires at a Mobil station. The attendants gave me a little gold bar that welcomed me to Greece, then with everything taken care of I was on my way. The shoreline was on my left most of the way. The clear waters of the Bay of Corinth reminded me of the stories I had read about Paul and his dedicated life.

By midafternoon the sky had turned dark and threatening. Speeding cars used the shoulder for a driving lane and constantly wanted me to move out of the way. Off-ramps were few and far between. What began as a drizzle soon turned into big drops of rain, and passing cars drenched me with waves of water.

It began to get dark and I needed to stop, both for safety reasons and because my body said so. I spotted a hotel and an off-ramp to get to it. I picked up my cycle and carried it up the winding stairs to my room on the second floor. (Sometimes the strength I had developed in my arms and legs surprised me.) A confections store and cafe across the street held a promise of supper, but crossing the road with its whizzing traffic provided a challenge, plus the marble in the paving mixture made the pavement very slippery, especially when wet. After I had spaghetti and tomato sauce in the cafe I returned to my room, thankful to still be in one piece. Although the shower was warm the room was cold, and I used a hot water bottle to warm the bed and help me relax into a peaceful sleep.

As I rode down the narrow roads into Corinth the next day, I saw a liberation, or holiday, celebration going on in town. The band played loudly and everything looked very festive. I thought of the apostle Paul again when I entered the city. He had walked these dusty streets more than 1,900 years before. The streets were paved now, but the hills and sea could not have changed that much.

Because it would not be necessary to cycle both ways, I decided to go from Corinth to Petra by train, then bike back to Corinth to take advantage of the westerly winds behind me. "Please be very careful with my bicycle," I begged the baggage handler. If my bicycle were damaged the delay could be disastrous.

I had a seat to myself. My socks and shirt hadn't gotten dry in the cold, damp hotel room the night before, so I put them on top of my bag to dry. I'd purchased some food at the supermarket, and now I could put my head back and chew away without a care in the world. The train stopped at little towns every few minutes, so it took two hours to go 90 miles. As we traveled I began organizing the stuff in my pockets. That's when I discovered that my inside jacket pocket really was not a pocket at all, and my precious mileage meter had disappeared. In Petra I was unsuccessfully trying to reach the train station in Corinth by phone when a young man, who had studied in America, came along. With his help we finally reached someone who said he would check around for the meter and let me know on Sunday when I arrived back in Corinth.

I learned from my travel brochure that Patras, with a population of 141,000 people, is the third-largest city in Greece. It stands below its Venetian castle on the site of the ancient city where, according to history, the apostle Andrew taught Christianity and was later crucified and buried. It is also from Patras that one sets out for Italy. It would have been nice to look around the famous city, but I needed to hurry on my way.

By 4:00, with my few belongings strapped on for safekeeping, I again faced east toward Athens. I had gone for miles without finding an off-ramp or exit into a village. My map indicated many small towns along the coast to my left, but I decided they must be on local roads along the shore. It was almost dark when I spotted a vine-covered house perched on the steep hillside. I lifted my bike over the guardrail and pushed it ahead of me up the rugged path. An older gentleman with a kind face stood in the front yard. I realized I faced all kinds of situations in these isolated areas, but I trusted God to stop me if what I was doing would get me into trouble. The man and I stood and looked across the lush tundra together as we enjoyed a quiet moment in that evening air. He told me there was a tunnel that would lead me to a small hotel down in the village across the road and gave me a note, telling them not to charge me more than L1000 (approximately US$8).

I don't know whether he had some ownership in the hotel, and I'm still wondering how I understood his Greek, but the place to which he directed me was a godsend. Since leaving at 4:00, I'd traveled 30 miles. The hotel would be a quiet place to rest on my day off. The room had no hot water and no heat, the blankets needed a good airing, and the water tasted musty. Still, I had a place to stay.

A rooster's crowing at 7:30 the next morning prompted me to wake up and get out of bed. A goat was bleating outside, dogs were barking, and hens were clucking. The backyard looked like a subtropical jungle. Lemon and grapefruit trees filled the neighbor's yard, and the hotel family had orange and banana trees. Green vines everywhere brightened the disarray.

That afternoon I sat quietly against the edge of the seawall, reading and watching the waves lapping against the shore. Nets draped over fishing boats dried in the sun, and children played near the shore while their mothers visited nearby. I might have lost my faith and courage and given up if it had not been for recalling some of the wonderful promises of the Bible that were jewels of strength when I needed them. One of my favorites has been "Trust in the Lord with all your heart, and do not rely on your own insight. In all your ways acknowledge him, and he will make straight your paths" (Prov. 3:5, 6, NRSV).

The next morning I loaded my bicycle and was traveling down the road by 7:20. The weather turned hot early, which surprised me in view of the cool nights. As more and more hills loomed ahead of me I adjusted the bicycle seat higher, tightened the left gears, and repositioned the left brake. By 11:30 I felt starved, and it didn't take long to put away the four oranges I had with me. They would have to sustain me until I found somewhere to stop for dinner.

The roads were very clean along the side, with few nails, but there was no shoulder for me to ride on, and several cars came too close for comfort. Still no sign of an off-ramp. I had clear sailing on the freeway and covered 50 miles, arriving near Corinth by 3:00.

When I studied the map later, I saw that, fortunately, I had taken the divided highway inland. An undivided road next to the Sea of Corinth serviced the many towns along the coast—I counted 34 towns between Egio and Corinth. The traffic on the narrow road by the sea would have probably delayed me.

If I felt hungry earlier in the day, now I was superstarved. I really wanted to find some vegetables and beans or legumes, but settled for apple juice, bread, a cone, and a cookie. It began to look as though great sections of the world had exchanged good old-fashioned food for junk. Candy bars and high-sugar, high-salt, high-calorie, high-fat, and low-nutritional-value foods were abundant along the thoroughfares that tourists used.

I decided to stay overnight at Hotel Belvue. I wanted to retrace some of the steps that the apostle Paul and his friends had made on their journeys in the first century. I struck up a conversation with a young girl from New York, who was trying to piece together a route that would take her over some of the paths of the past. After I left my bike at the hotel we boarded a bus and took off together.

When we reached Corinth, we took a taxi to the top of the hill. A great walled fortification, built to withstand the battles and storms of time, stood near the top. We saw the place where Paul was supposed to have preached to the Grecians about the risen Christ. Walking around the old city encouraged me to be a better Christian and to grasp, even a little, Paul's complete dedication to the cause he believed in.

Back in my room that night I noticed dark red blotches all over the walls. Squashed mosquitoes. And as soon as I turned out the lights their surviving friends attacked in full force. I was being eaten alive. All night I kept turning on the tiny light that hung in the middle of the room so I could kill the invaders resting on the wall. Losing a little blood was not the issue—mosquitoes can carry serious diseases such as encephalitis and malaria. The next morning I looked like I'd developed chicken pox. (As long as I'm complaining I might as well mention the bed that sank in the middle like a bathtub, the bathroom that was down the hall and around the corner, and the cold air and cold water in the room.

Invigorating, and definitely helpful in encouraging me to get dressed quickly and get away from the hotel next morning.)

I asked about my mileage meter at the train station. No one gave me a glimmer of hope that it would be found. I knew I'd miss it and had no idea how long it would be until I could get another one. It was so much easier to monitor my speed and the distance traveled with a meter. If I ever got another one I vowed I would never let it out of my sight! (Gene did send me a replacement, but it never reached me.)

Since I'd already ridden to Corinth, I got back on the train to Piraeus. (If I were to do it again I think it would be easier to either land in Patras and ride to Athens, or go all the way on the train and ride my bike back to Athens.) I arrived in Piraeus, still 20 miles or so from where the girls lived in Athens and where I'd left some of my things until I returned. It was getting warmer now, and I wanted to box up my down coat and some other items and ship them home.

Once on my way to Athens I wondered if I'd be able to find the apartment. Nobody on a bicycle is eager to wade through exhaust fumes, noise, and speeding drivers in a big city, only to find themselves right back where they started. Relief washed over me when I recognized the tree-lined lane and the porch of the girls' upstairs apartment. They had worked until 3:00 a.m. and were still in bed when I arrived. It took me quite a while to rearrange everything and pack what I was not taking with me. Carol said she'd take care of sending the box home for me. By 5:00 my panniers were clicked in place on the front and back wheels of the bicycle. I said goodbye and started for the airport, thankful that I'd conquered my first milepost across the lower peninsula of Greece.

The plane landed in Tel Aviv about 8:30 that evening. I wondered how cycling and walking along the Mediterranean Sea would compare to the Sea of Corinth. I took a taxi to the hotel, where a hot soak in the tub and a comfortable bed made the day complete. The next day Sarah Cohen in the Ministry of Tourism office promised to do everything possible to help me plan the next move.

THE PROMISED LAND

Before setting out, I had the bicycle checked, tightening the brake and some other nuts and bolts that rattled a little. As I headed for a hostel farther north, I noticed uniformed soldiers (both men and women) everywhere. Most were waiting for rides home from military school, and people were stopping to pick them up. At the hostel I was assigned to the newer of two buildings. A river ran close by, and subtropical plants grew inside and outside in an atmosphere of relaxation and acceptance.

That evening I spoke on the phone with Pastor Ermanno Garbi, president of the Seventh-day Adventist conference in Jerusalem. Pastor Garbi and I had planned to go to Jerusalem, but because of the unrest in the city I had been advised to cancel the trip. The pastor, however, was very eager that I come, and as we talked I felt impressed that I must go, even though this trip was not part of my riding route. I'd have to come back to Tel Aviv and go north from there.

The Garbis are a lovely couple. After dinner in their home, he drove me to the office of the Jerusalem *Post*. The newspaper, printed in English, has a worldwide circulation. Herb, a young journalist, seemed fascinated by my story and took numerous pictures as he interviewed me for an hour. When the article and picture (which took up 27 column inches) came out in the magazine section of the *Post,* Herb sent a copy to Gene back home.

Gene told a friend, "When I opened the paper, there was Mom, as big as life, with her AROUND THE WORLD banner shouting at me and her message of hope and health beaming into the airways, even as the picture was being taken. I'm just glad she's still alive!"

The pastor needed to go to Tel Aviv, so he offered me a ride back to my hotel. On the way he pointed out the names of hills and other landmarks made famous by stories of Jesus and the apostles. We passed a small cable car stopped on the tracks on a steep hill not far from the city. The occupants had been fired on and killed as they carried supplies across the hills, the pastor said.

The next day was the last day of March, and I was eager to get out of the hustle and bustle of the city. I experienced a little anxiety crossing the bridge in the traffic, but soon I was on my way. I seemed to be constantly climbing as I rode. A strong west wind, blowing off the Mediterranean Sea, cooled me a little, but it was tough cycling through some of the high places. After a brief stop for lunch I was on the road again. A heavy crosswind hit the panniers with such force that I had to walk and push my bike. Two ladies stopped and asked what I was doing. When I told them about my mission and my goal they seemed interested, saying they enjoyed cycling, and promised to write to me.

Toward evening the dust faded away, but it was still tough going. The previous evening I had phoned Pastor Vebersax and his wife, who lived on top of Mount Carmel in Haifa. They expected me sometime during the day. As I stood at the foot of the mountain, wondering where to go next, I noticed a woman nearby. She appeared to be waiting for someone or something. When I told her that Pastor Vebersax was expecting me, I discovered that he lived on the same block that she did! She phoned him for me and offered to take me to his house. We put my bike in the trunk of her car and started up the very steep grade, which was quite a climb even for a car. I felt a sense of awe. This was the same mountain Elijah had climbed when the 400 prophets of Baal couldn't get their gods to send fire from heaven to burn their sacrifices.

Before I left the next morning, I felt I must sit down and finish my report for the people back home. Telling where I'd been and where I was going usually took about 10 hand-written pages. I labeled the pictures that accompanied the copy for the press. I appreciated the pastor's offer to mail the package for me as this task sometimes resulted in a delay. I wanted to get to Capernaum before the Sabbath.

On my way to Capernaum I saw a sign that pointed to Caesarea, another historical landmark in the life of Jesus. This was desert, and a hot east wind did its best to stop me in my tracks. At times I could scarcely push the bicycle. Prevailing winds are usually from the west, but that day they changed, bringing dust and heat from farther inland. I ate a lot of dust because it was hard to keep my mouth shut—I needed maximum oxygen to keep going. I stopped to rest on a little ledge jutting out from the rock wall, offering about two feet of shade beside the cliff. The sun beat almost straight down on me. Traffic was light, and there were no settlements nearby. Not even a rabbit ventured out in the noonday sun! The wind finally died down about 3:00. As I got closer to Tiberias, the fields became greener. Grains and other plants flourished, thanks to an irrigation system. The desert had indeed turned into a garden paradise.

A steep, downhill grade to the Sea of Galilee and Tiberias had me wondering if I might not go right over the handlebars if I didn't watch my speed. I stopped at the police station at the bottom of the hill and called Simo Perko, the pastor from Nazareth, who offered to come and pick me up.

Not sure just what to do next, I asked him if I should go on to Capernaum and complete the journey, or come back on Sunday. Since it wouldn't take long to finish, he followed behind me and shone the car lights on the road so I could see where I was riding. The cool evening air refreshed me and new energy seeped into my bones. We reached the city gates of Capernaum about 7:00. They were locked. We stood quietly, listening to the night sounds, lost in our own thoughts. On this night nearly 2,000 years before, Jesus had rested in a borrowed tomb.

After breakfast the next morning, Mrs. Perko, their two children, and I walked down to the Health and Evangelistic Center in the city of Nazareth. It was hot and dusty, and piles of garbage lay everywhere. (Apparently the garbage pick-up department was on strike.) Droves of flies dominated the scene, and it looked discouraging at best. Many of the people seemed sad and frustrated.

I spoke during the church service. Nagib Khoury, a teacher in Nazareth, served as my interpreter. He'd been in the Liberation League in 1947-1948. Sometimes I feel I have been sheltered from difficult experiences that are commonplace in the lives of those who have always lived in an atmosphere of conflict.

After dinner we climbed a high hill to Nain, where Jesus had restored life to a widow's son even as the funeral procession made its way to the cemetery. I gave a talk to a group of Muslim children, who then sang some of their songs for me.

The next day Simo and his family took me to the airport in Tel Aviv. I had to return to Athens and would fly to Karachi from there. (Israel and Pakistan were not on good terms at the time.) In Athens I visited the Acropolis, or sacred rock, once more. The magnificence of the Parthenon is almost beyond comprehension. I walked through those immense columns that have stood there for 500 years. No one knows how they were raised into place. Although we have come up with many great inventions, and travel today seems to reach for the stars, some secrets buried with time leave many questions unanswered.

THE LONGEST DAY OF MY LIFE

I loaded the panniers on the bike, filled my water bottles, checked the tires, then put on my helmet and gloves and pointed my wheels out into a new world. It was about 15 miles to Karachi, and the road by the airport looked well paved; busy, but not confusing. I'd heard that the Metropole Hotel in Karachi wasn't too expensive, so off I went with a silent prayer for protection.

Before long I hit heavy traffic. Passengers jammed the open-air buses with people hanging out every window and door. The buses pulled into stops, then quickly moved back into the street. I just hoped one wouldn't land on top of me. Within minutes, two motorbikes flanked me on either side; one was so close I gestured for him to move over so he wouldn't hit me. As we rode along, both riders kept firing questions at me.

"What's your name?"

"Why are you riding a bicycle?"

"Where are you going?"

"How old are you?"

"Where are you from?"

As Pakistani women do not ride bikes, I received a lot of attention from all sides. Jitneys, carts, taxis, buses, and people jammed the streets. Most travelers who weren't on tours rode the trains and buses and stayed in the hostels. I seldom saw a cyclist touring the country for the fun of it.

Once I reached the hotel I bathed, then sank down on the bed and slept for three hours. The room, though not spotless, was air-conditioned, which helped me get some much-needed rest. About 4:00 I went out on the streets. The sight of beggars, some of them crippled little children, pained my heart. They sat on the street hour after hour in the heat and stench with just a newspaper (or sometimes nothing at all) under them. Everyone dressed in a similar style—baggy pants and a tunic. It seemed their clothing had come from the same bolt of cloth and had been cut from the same simple pattern.

In a small restaurant I ordered tomato soup and a whole-wheat bun. Both tasted wonderful and helped to restore my energy. By the time I left the restaurant dusk had arrived. I walked rapidly, very much aware that I was alone in the dark in a strange city, and it didn't take me long to reach the hotel. What if I had gotten lost? I knew I must be more careful in the future.

The next day I decided to visit the American Embassy to find out about travel conditions in Pakistan. After I stated what I was doing, a woman frisked me and sent me into a waiting room. While I waited, the press interviewed me. Then a security officer checked me over again to be sure I wasn't there to cause trouble. Eventually, the regional security officer, R. A. Deibler, came out to talk to me. I told him of my concern over an article in the morning paper that stated the north border was closed and that there had been 100 deaths in nine days.

He confirmed the report. "Do not go up there on a bicycle. A band of Eacoits is going right through there," he warned me. "These bandits have a home base near Lahore and have kidnapped, robbed, and killed people, and even shot at cars on the road. No, it is not safe, even with a guide."

I'd heard many warnings of doom and death before, but this one had a little more bite in it. I walked around town for an hour, watching where I went so I could find my way back to the hotel. Masses of humanity, mostly men, milled around me everywhere.

The Muslim faith does not allow men and women together on the same streets. I saw boys and men wherever I looked, holding hands, and apparently going nowhere. Groups of women filled the yardage shops, where shop owners shouted for customers to come look at their goods. The overall impression was one of bedlam.

The heat, the smell of streets used for years as bathrooms, the mud, filth, piles of rubble, and the jostling crowds began to wear on my nerves. How must it be for those who are locked in this environment? I turned my ankle during my walk, and the pain was getting worse. I decided to return to the hotel before I became lost.

The hotel clerk said a gentleman had called and asked for me. Earlier in the day I'd asked a man on the street if he could tell me how to find the airline office. He'd immediately hailed a cab, got in, and motioned for me to follow. I hesitated, but he was well-dressed and we were right in the city, so I did. He waited in the cab while I was in the airline office, then brought me back to the hotel. He'd been very friendly, and now it appeared he wanted to become better acquainted. I knew I must find another place to stay. But right then I needed more sleep. I prayed that God would let me know what to do and soon drifted off to sleep in the cool air. My ankle was quite painful during the night, but felt better the next morning.

I decided a town this size must have someplace I could stay—a mission, church, or hospital. I looked in the yellow pages and almost shouted with relief. In fact, the people at Karachi Adventist Hospital had been expecting my arrival. Austin, the health educator, had planned an itinerary for me! Just as I was about to get into his truck, my taxi-hailing friend from the hotel showed up and pleaded with me to allow him to get to know me better. I assured him I would be well cared for at the mission and thanked him for his help.

Although the hospital could use some help in updating and remodeling, the staff is doing a wonderful service in taking care of the large number or patients who daily passed through their doors. My dear friends, Robert and Ann Dunn, had founded Karachi Adventist Hospital 40 years before. He later served as the physician in our FRESH START for Health program at Andrews University, and Ann helped with some of the programs. They raised nine children and devoted much of their lives to helping others regain, or retain, their health.

When we arrived at the hospital compound, a staff member showed me to an upstairs apartment belonging to a mission teacher who was out on an assignment. It felt wonderful to have a place to relax. That evening I spoke to about 40 student nurses. After the meeting Austin invited me to his home to meet his wife, Jeannie, and their five children. Jeannie had prepared a tasty supper and served papaya ice cream for dessert.

The next morning I ate breakfast with the Fowlers, a family from Salmon Arm, British Columbia, who lived in the apartment below me. Amazing! Here I was on the other side of the world, enjoying breakfast with a family whose home was less than an hour's drive from where I had been born!

I finished my letters home, then sent two letters and a telegram to India regarding my arrival the next week. After dinner I joined long lines of people at the post office, waiting in the hot, sultry air for their turn at the window. The smell was hard to handle, although a number of the hospital staff said one eventually becomes used to it.

It was indeed a blessing to be at the hospital. I'd hoped to head north before long, but the extra days were a godsend for my sunburned lips and my cold. So was the good food and purified water. I would need all the help I could get before entering the Punjab.

My time of rest and recreation ended. Austin, who was also going to Lahore, would get me safely on the train. From Lahore I would cycle to a private school in the Punjab. The train was a scene of mass confusion. Austin had to go into a separate car with the rest of the men, leaving me to try and get to my seat. The second-class cars were full, so I opted for third-class. There were so many people on the train that it was difficult to walk down the aisle. Everyone competed for a place to sit. Hoisting my bike up onto the wooden shelf above, I wedged in among six people on a bench and laid my head back to try to get a little sleep.

The whistle blew and the train stopped at every four-corner intersection. People threw orange peels and everything else on the floor or out the open window. The toilet, a hole flush with the floor, occupied one corner of a small room. As the train jerked back and forth down the track, negotiating a squatting position in order to perform one's bodily functions required physical fitness of the highest caliber. Of course, there was no toilet paper or water for washing hands. That had to be the longest day of my life. I promised myself that night that I would never complain again about anything. Maybe this is where I first got diarrhea. Although I didn't get sick, it didn't help.

The next morning Austin came by to tell me it would be another 11 or 12 hours before we'd arrive in Lahore. We'd already been on the train since 9:30 the night before, but complaining wouldn't help. I couldn't get out and walk, so I decided to take things as they were.

The train passed scattered villages of family homes surrounded by mud-and-brick walls. Animals filled the compounds. Often I saw people living in shacks. Vendors shouted at each of the train's frequent stops, each one trying to sell his wares. I wanted a cold drink but dared not take a chance on the water. The passengers were kind and friendly and the children well-behaved, sitting for hours without complaining. When a woman offered me her top bunk, I gratefully accepted and slept for several hours on the hard bench of open slats. When the whistle finally sounded at the end of the line, there could not have been a happier passenger getting off the train than I.

A Mr. Smith, returning to the Seventh-day Adventist Pakistan Union Mission, rode with me in a three-wheeler that I hired to take us to the compound. The Collier family, who were from England, invited me to spend the night with them. Pastor Collier was away on business, but Mrs. Collier welcomed me. Their daughter, who was somewhat of a tomboy, reminded me of myself 50 years before. We enjoyed a pleasant evening together, and I knew that I'd remember these special times when the going was tough. In the morning I'd be out on the road on my bicycle. In the meantime, I enjoyed one more night of peaceful rest.

I planned to visit in the Sheikhpura District, west of Lahore.

There had been some internal rumblings in the Punjab, and I hoped the bandits would not decide to move into the area. David Shana, a clean-cut young man with a wife and two young children, worked at the mission as the gardener. His sister lived about halfway between Lahore and the seminary (a title used for private schools). I felt very blessed when I learned that David would accompany me to the school and then back to Lahore. We would stop at his sister's home to rest during the trip.

We paid 130 rupees to have a taxi take us and our bicycles to the edge of the city. As we bicycled through the countryside, great clouds of dust from the powdery soil filled the air. The masses of humanity along the way defied description. The ground around the village water pumps was thick with mud. Water buffalo wallowed in little mud ponds or stood on short tethers tied to trees. Sheep, goats, and mules crowded the road and the yards. Donkeys and Brahman cows pulled carts or carried heavy loads on their backs.

We'd traveled only a short distance when one of David's bicycle tires went flat. It was 18 kilometers to the nearest bicycle repair shop. I knew I'd have to go on alone; David could catch up with me later. A truck hauling hay offered him a ride to the shop. He wanted me to accompany him since he'd received strict instructions at the mission to take good care of me. But I told him I felt I had to keep going, and he went on without me.

However, the hay truck had barely gotten out of sight when I saw a man on the side of the road fixing bicycles. So did a much-relieved David. I bought a new tire for his bicycle, and we waited for the man to put it on. Within seconds a crowd of men and boys gathered around me. Most them were dressed in the usual white suit with baggy pants and looked very comfortable in the heat. A tall, gray-haired man crossed the road and spoke to me in English. I gathered he was the village patriarch. He asked where I was going and why. I explained my mission.

David watched anxiously as more men and boys joined the crowd that began to press in around me. I finally told him I was going to ride on slowly, and he could catch up with me when the tire was on his bicycle. The crowd parted, allowing me to pass without any trouble. As soon as I was out on the road again, a young man appeared a short distance in front of me, riding a bicycle that sported colored streamers hanging from the handlebars. Both his clothes and his bicycle were clean, but I wasn't sure of his intentions and hesitated to ride too close to him. We didn't exchange any words, and I doubt we would have understood each other if we had. When I stopped on a bridge to let him get farther ahead, he also stopped and waited until I began to move again. He stayed right in front of me until David arrived, then rode off ahead of us. I wondered if perhaps the village patriarch had sent him to guard me.

As we rode along, the blowing horns, dust, exhaust fumes, and heat seemed overpowering, in spite of the mask I wore. When we stopped at a bridge so that David could take a picture, the sudden stop after riding faster than usual in the extreme heat caused me to nearly faint. I quickly put my head between my knees and the danger passed. David became alarmed and suggested that we didn't need to continue. He soon discovered that I wasn't one to give up easily. We rode slower after that, and I had no more trouble.

About 3:00 David announced we had arrived at his sister's village. The town was off the main road and most of the homes were surrounded by walls. When we entered the swept-clean courtyard inside the walls around his sister's home, I felt as though we were in our own little world. A few chickens pecked away at anything that seemed edible, and a little white dog wandered aimlessly around the yard. A separate building housed the bathroom, which had water in a pail for flushing the toilet. There were no screens on the front of the house to discourage the ubiquitous flies, and the entrance to the kitchen and bedrooms needed a new screen door. (I gave Lab, the grandfather, 250 rupees to help with the new door.) Because of the thick walls surrounding them, these inner rooms were cooler.

Lab had suffered a heart attack some months earlier and had become quite overweight and inactive. I encouraged him to move about more and to use less oil in the cooking. He was a kind man and still needed by his family. I felt he could hope again if he would only walk each day facing the sunrise, instead of waiting for the sun to go down in his life.

David's sister did everything she could to make me feel welcome. She prepared rice, vegetables, and several other dishes that she set before us. The heat had taken away some of my usual enthusiasm for food, but I did eat a little, then rested on one of the beds before we were once more on our way.

We arrived at the school around 5:00. The school was so close to the road that we could still hear the blowing horns and traffic noises, but the lovely trees shaded us from the sun. David returned to his sister's home for the night, but would be back the next morning to accompany me on the ride back to Lahore.

I had supper with Dr. Deo and Karen Fieber from the United States. The tangerine drink they served was the best I've ever tasted. It looked like the tangerines had been put in the blender, then the juice and pulp mixture frozen and served as a drink.

That evening I spoke to 400 elementary and high school students at their evening worship hour. The students, all wearing uniforms, looked happy and healthy. I spent the night with Dr. and Mrs. Hedley Eager, who had been at Andrews University when I taught there. They had come to Pakistan as missionaries. Although we weren't far from the large ammunition dump that had blown up a few weeks earlier, I had no fear. My heavenly Friend was still along on the ride.

David arrived about 9:45 the next morning and we set out. The day soon became as sweltering hot as the one before had been. I told myself to just continue to put one leg down and the other up, watch for obstacles in my path, and surely we would reach Lahore eventually. We stopped at David's sister's home for lunch. The heat had taken my appetite away, and even though my system needed the energy I just couldn't eat very much of her bountiful spread.

After a brief rest I knew we must get back on the road. An occasional roadside tree offered a little shade as we passed. Whenever we stopped to rest, even for a few seconds, people gathered around us. By the time we reached the outskirts of Lahore at 4:30, we'd traveled 52 kilometers. David bargained for a jitney taxi that gave us a very bumpy ride to the mission station. I was dirty, my hair was stiff, and my body a mixture of sweat and dust. But after I cleaned up and cooled off, my appetite returned. When bedtime arrived I sincerely hoped the mosquitoes were on vacation.

The next day I interviewed with a journalist from a health magazine that circulated among 520 colleges in the country. In the afternoon one of the teachers and I visited a family out in the country where I had the opportunity to learn more about the customs and culture of the region. High walls completely surrounded the family compound. The whole place was neat and swept clean. A long structure inside the compound was divided into seven sections with doors in front. Shelves covered with embroidered runners filled the back walls of the small rooms. Each couple in the family had goblets and other dishes that had been given to them on their wedding day lined up on the shelves. Little birds that flew in and out had also built their homes inside. Outside the structure, girls squatted in front of individual stoves on which cooking pots bubbled over an opening in the stove top. They added sticks to the fire from another opening in front.

Everyone was neatly dressed in the usual light-colored baggy pants. Family members of all ages, from babies to the elderly, moved around the compound. Just inside the gate, quite a distance from the house, several animals were tethered in one corner of a small enclosure that was open on one end. A narrow ditch, serving as a latrine, had been dug in the ground. I was told that the women must go out into the fields for defecation, either before sunrise or after dark. They train themselves to this schedule while very young. The men are allowed to go whenever the need arises.

I shall always be grateful for that short visit. It showed me how very, very simple life can be. The family members have time to spend with each other; they do not need things to be happy. I contrasted their life with the TV shows back home depicting power, the desire for material possessions, crime, lying, stealing, adultery, and broken homes. I felt downcast when I thought of the example my country often broadcasts to the world.

On our way back to the mission we stopped to watch a man

make chapati. A small fire burned inside a round cylinder in the ground. He cooked small, flat, whole-wheat cakes on the hot sides of the cylinder.

Pastor Collier returned home that evening and told us about his trip into the interior. Someone had blown up a large stockpile of ammunition, and although one of the bombs had gone through the roof of a pastor's home, no one had been hurt.

The next morning it was time to pack and leave for the airport. Bicycle time spent on the road in Pakistan had been brief, but I hoped I could make up some miles farther along in my trip. If the adventures I'd encountered in Pakistan were any indication of what lay ahead, I knew I was in for more surprises.

We touched down in Delhi, India, a 2:30. As I stood in the airport I remembered the advice of a travel agent back home who had been born and raised in India. "Don't go through India on a bike," she warned me. "Food and water problems are bad enough, but consider being robbed of everything you have. Those people are poor, and they will not hesitate to harm you to get what you have. You could contract a gastric-intestinal infection and be left out there to die, and no one back home would be the wiser!"

Now here I was in this country teeming with millions of people who were poor and needed what I had. I knew I would have never come if I'd not been convinced this was what I was supposed to do. I trusted God to take care of me just as He had in every other situation. I knew every angel in heaven would be sent to help me, if necessary.

WELCOME, CHARLOTTE HAMLIN! read the big sign on the road to the conference center. When I walked in, missionaries from Singapore were looking at a copy of *Focus*, a magazine sent to Andrews University alumni all over the world. The page they were looking at had a picture of me and an article about my trip around the world.

We all piled into a bus to do a little sightseeing. We visited the beautiful Bahai House of Worship, an oasis in an otherwise drab existence. Dedicated to God, the auditorium of the temple is open to all for prayer and meditation, regardless of race, nation, caste, class, or creed. Just across the street I witnessed the lowest of human lifestyles. People used pieces of board and paper to make shacks for shelter. Communal crowding opened the way for disease and filth of every kind.

We visited the grounds where Mrs. Ghandi had been so tragically assassinated. Large windows around her office area allowed visitors to get a glimpse of how things had been left at the time of her death. Our next stop was the eternal flame memorial of Mahatma Ghandi, another rare human being, who thought only of others and gave all he had for them.

That night I enjoyed a meal of baked beans and instant mashed potatoes. To my way of thinking right then, it was a feast. Bedtime brought another battle with the mosquitoes. I had a choice. If I left the overhead fan running all night, it was noisy and stirred up the dust, but the wind from the fan discouraged the mosquitoes. If I turned it off the mosquitoes had a clear field of attack. I decided to let the fan run.

I ate breakfast with Dr. Baglien, who worked at the compound. Although paralyzed on one side, she managed to walk slowly along. She'd had a brain tumor, then a stroke, followed by a broken hip. Her husband, also employed by the mission and often away in the field, had a retina detachment requiring surgery. In spite of the difficulties in her life she was cheerful and invited me to share some meals with her. I realized I had very little about which to complain.

While in Delhi, I took a bus to the Taj Mahal—a long day's trip. The highway we traveled was absolute chaos. Wrecked trucks, buses, and other vehicles littered the middle and each side of the highway. One couldn't be sure which side of an obstacle another vehicle would choose to take. Sometimes we couldn't see what was coming from the other way. Most of the time, our driver drove on the wrong side of the road.

Before I left Delhi I visited the marketplace and purchased some nice-looking mangoes. What a letdown when I tried to eat them! They'd been picked green in order to get them to market early, then artificially ripened. I shopped for a pair of lightweight sandals in an alley shoe store. Someone threw shoes down to the clerk through a hole in the ceiling. This method was actually efficient and fast.

Dr. Baglien had made me promise I'd visit the U.S. Embassy before I left Delhi. The regional security officer (who was from Detroit, only a four-hour drive from my home in Michigan) advised me to try to get to Moradabad by 4:30 p.m.

"They've been having some demonstrations and riots there," she told me. "Otherwise, you should be perfectly safe. It would be best to have someone with you, but I feel you'll be all right on the road." Her positive words were a great encouragement. I knew God was my mainstay and Friend, but we all need a little human confirmation now and then.

After a visit to the Nepalese embassy for a visa, I mailed my documentaries and pictures home, packed my bags, and was ready to leave early the next morning.

RESCUED BY A MESSENGER

Pastor S. P. Chand, president of the Upper Ganges and Hapur District, had been most cooperative in arranging my stay in Delhi. He also arranged for two men to accompany me out of Delhi until I was safely headed east toward Hapur. When we started out at 5:45, it was cool with little traffic so early on a Sunday morning. However, when we arrived at the edge of any village we found crowded roads and shops. It took care and skill to weave in and out without being hit by trucks, or anything or anyone else, going anywhere they chose to go. It was quite an oddity to be on a road with few rules. Everywhere I looked trucks and buses lay on their sides or completely upside-down. Animals had the free run of the road. Dogs weren't too much of a threat—they were so thin and undernourished that they walked, not ran.

The two men accompanied me about 15 of the 32 miles to Hapur. We stopped at an intersection in the road, where they planned to return by a different route. When a crowd began to gather I asked the men to come with me just a little farther so that the crowd would not see me traveling on alone. Before they had to turn back, we prayed together and shook hands. Then suddenly they were gone. That alone feeling started to creep over me. Women don't ride bikes in India. How would men accept my presence on the road?

I began to pedal rapidly, eager to get more miles behind me. Women along the roadside were making dung cakes for fuel by mixing dung from buffalo and other animals with straw before patting them into round cakes and stacking them in the shape of a beehive to dry.

At the beginning of our journey that morning we'd seen the police and a number of onlookers surround a body at the side of the road. The dead man had been traveling in the night. I remembered the warning not to travel on the road after dark.

Occasionally, small trees dotted the landscape, but the grass looked brown and dry, even though it was April. Sometimes larger trees lined the road on both sides and I enjoyed riding along in their shade. That little bit of cooler air helped tremendously. Every time I stopped, even momentarily, a crowd would gather. So I tried to stop when few people were on the road and before a village came into view.

As I neared Hapur I began to wonder how anyone would be able to find me in that mass of moving people. I hoped someone would spot me by my helmet. And they did! Several men from the Adventist mission, where a large school is located, had come out to the main road to meet me. As I stepped into the rickshaw for the trip into town, one of my carrier frames that held the front pannier fell apart. Evidently I had lost a nut and bolt as I traveled. What would I have done if this had happened while I was out on the road?

Pastor Chand, his wife, and two daughters welcomed me into their home. It felt good to visit with this family around their table and to have a room for the night. By 6:30 the next morning I was on the road to Moradabad. I hoped to arrive by 4:30. Curiosity seekers followed me all day. One very thin fellow stayed too close for comfort. When I stopped by the side of the road to see if he would continue on, he became angry and motioned for me to move along. Then when he saw me drink from my water bottle his scowl turned to a broad grin. As I started down the road again I wondered what my next move should be. Eventually I came to a downhill grade, not steep, but with enough incline for me to get into a lower gear and outrun him. I didn't see him again until I reached a village far down the road. He didn't try to follow me.

Loudspeakers blared as I passed through several villages. Groups of people gathered under tents for some kind of meeting. Now and then I heard the word "America." I began to hope that Moradabad was not too far away. I'd be a good target if the crowds decided to vent their feelings. When a group from the school came out to meet me, I felt very thankful and relieved to see them standing by the road. The principal, B. M. Jawath, welcomed me. "We are very happy to meet you, and we wish you a very safe journey. May God protect you."

I replied with a short talk about the journey I was making and what I wanted to accomplish. I emphasized living a healthy lifestyle so we can enjoy each day as it comes along. Though life is not easy, it's much more pleasant when we feel good and can do the things that give us pleasure in our homes and travels.

I'd gone 46.6 miles for the day. Not a record, but it had answered my biggest concern: It might be tough at times, but I could make it in India.

Children began to arrive before I left the next morning. The school population included 1,000 students from different Christian persuasions. Three employees accompanied me to the bridge, and then I was on my own again. As the bike covered mile after mile, I continued to draw the attention of people along the way. I couldn't really blame them. I did look a little strange with fabric attached to my touring shorts to cover my legs, and with cut-off sleeves on my arms.

By midmorning I began to pray for somewhere to stop. Hungry, hot, and miserable from the dry, dusty road, I needed a place to rest for a while. My prayers were answered when I saw a sign for the Methodist Mission by the edge of the road. The pastor and his family welcomed me to the mission and seemed fascinated by the canned heat I used to prepare my meal. I added some hot water to dried potatoes and made mashed potatoes while the beans I had bought boiled away in the pot. I hoped the ever-present swarm of flies land-ing everywhere wouldn't contaminate them. Some chapatis com-pleted my meal. The family left me alone to eat my food and take a quick siesta. I returned to the road feeling refreshed.

I had the address of the Gould family, my contact in Bareilly. When I stopped at a medical office for directions, they sent a young man with me to find the place. We went up a steep stairway to an outer court, then to a long, one-story house at the other end. They were expecting me, and I appreciated the opportunity to be clean again and enjoy a meal with the family around the table and to be able to spend the night with them. I made 59 miles that day and was indeed in the interior of India where the people lived and the tourists didn't come.

The next day I pedaled from Bareilly to the outskirts of Shahjahanpur. I saw the Lapwing motel and restaurant, operated by the U.P. State Tourism Development Corporation, and decided to spend the night, hoping they might serve food I could eat. All rooms opened onto a veranda. (That was good.) The water cooler seemed loaded with mildew or mold of some kind. (That was bad. My nose started to stop up almost immediately.)

I needed to cash a traveler's check and hurried to the State Bank of India down the street. The clerk put me in a room piled high with papers and worn counters. "Sit down in front of this desk," he instructed.

The room didn't look as if it had anything to do with a bank, but then I didn't exactly look like Cinderella either. Men began en-tering the room and, before many minutes passed, bank personnel lined up against three walls. Apparently nobody wanted to miss the drama unfolding in front of them.

"Is it possible for me to cash a $100 travelers check?" I directed my question to the room at large.

"The State Bank of India cannot do that," one of the men replied. "You must come back tomorrow, and we will take you to a money exchange place."

"Tomorrow is the day I go to church," I said. "I cannot do business then."

How much they understood of what I said remains a mystery. I finally went outside where I discovered several men examining my bicycle, trying out the gears, and wondering about the soft jell-like seat. Concerned that they might damage something, I quickly left. Back at the hotel, I tried to tell the waiter I couldn't drink anything but boiled water and could eat only cooked food that was hot. Despite my efforts, the rice was served cold. I knew I shouldn't eat it but was so hungry that I went against my better judgment. That night I went to sleep with only ten cents in my pocket. There was no point in staying awake to worry about it. I did have a roof over my head, and my Partner was along and would take care of things.

The next day I phoned the Shri Ram Chandra Mission-Ashram. Yes, I could stay there. Some boys on the street gave me directions, and before long I arrived. Rasiklal Kanjee, of Indian descent but born in South Africa, took me into the temple and explained their program. Volunteers did everything. For one hour in the morning, he said, everyone sat on the floor in the temple to meditate and pray. They returned in the evening for another hour to review the day and take care of any wrongs or make needed changes.

Saturday evening I couldn't eat. Nausea overwhelmed me and I had diarrhea. Everyone was sitting cross-legged on the floor in the kitchen, eating the fried vegetables with their hands. I would have liked to join them, but went to my room instead. It was too hot to use even a sheet, so I decided to sleep in a tunic and trousers made from fairly light material. I felt this looked modest enough in India where women covered both their legs and head. I left the door and shutters open to encourage any little current of moving air. At dusk the mosquitoes swarmed through the window.

That evening Rasiklal and I had a long talk. I told him what it meant to be a Christian and that I believed Jesus was the Son of God, not just a prophet. He spoke about several of his beliefs. I also met M. D. Jahagirdar, the chief circuit judge of Bangalore, India. The city supplied three guards to ensure his safety. M. S. Kodagall, a contractor, was also anxious about my welfare. He went into town to get me some ice cubes and bought me some grapes. All the attention embarrassed me, but not so much that I would exchange it for the open road! I'm sure they didn't know much about the Ten Commandments, but they lived closer to the lifestyle of the Man from Galilee than many who claim to know Him.

That night they gave me a mosquito net, but I didn't put it up properly and one arm hung out from under the netting. The next morning I counted 20 mosquito bites on the back of my upper arm. I prayed that none of the mosquitoes carried malaria. I really wasn't interested in doing research to see if the medicine I'd taken worked.

I'd planned to leave at 8:00 the next morning, but slept on hour after hour. People came and went all day. The nausea lessened, but I'd eaten very little. Rasiklal brought me some herbs and medicine. Somehow I knew it was all right to take them. I had some antibiotics with me, but wanted to keep them in case of an emergency. After eating gruel the kitchen staff prepared, I did feel a little stronger. I washed some clothes and hung them around the room to dry, praying that tomorrow would be a better day.

Sharad Chandra, grandson of the mission's founder, came by Sunday evening. We talked about world events and everyday things. He'd just married an educated young bride, and they were very happy. He told me his faith was not popular in India—someone had poisoned him six months earlier. He survived but was still very weak. Sharad was in charge of the work at the mission and felt the responsibility of his position. He invited me to stay as long as necessary, urging me to come and stay with him and his wife at the other end of the compound. (His palace had 42 rooms.) He'd heard about the Bank of India refusing to exchange my travelers checks and pulled a roll of money from his pocket.

"I will be glad to exchange your traveler's checks for you," he said.

I was still weak the next morning. They begged me to stay another day to get my strength back, but I felt that I must go on. I shall always be thankful for that experience. I felt safe and cared for at a time when it would have been impossible for me to continue on the road.

Two hours down the road, I had to stop and rest. Three

teenage boys came by, standing and staring at me as I chewed away on a piece of bread. Then rain began to fall. An elderly man stood near a lean-to outside the gate to a family compound. I indicated with gestures that I wanted to get out of the rain, and he waved for me to come over to the lean-to. He placed a much-used pad on a cot and I collapsed on it, taking deep gasps of air, trying to relax. The old man sat by me with a big fan, driving the flies away from my face, while his wife boiled some water for me on a little stove. I thanked God for the opportunity to lie there, close my eyes, and catch my breath, and for these people who helped a stranger in distress. Finally I felt able to resume my journey.

Later that day it rained again. I stopped at a gas station and laid on a cot indoors until the sky cleared. An hour before sunset I knew I wouldn't get to Sitapur before dark. Someone had told me there were no accommodations before Sitapur, and I knew it would be suicide to be on the road after dark. When I inquired of several farmers about a place to stay, they only shook their heads. I should have listened to the people back at the temple grounds. I finally decided I couldn't just stand there on the side of the road. I rode on, going northeast, leaving everything in God's care.

Suddenly a young man, clean-shaven and well-groomed, wearing a cream-colored suit, rode up beside me on his bicycle. Addressing me in English, he talked as we rode along the road together. I asked if he knew where I might spend the night.

"Why, yes," he said. "In Mahoba, just up the road about 15 kilometers, is a PWD inspection guest house for officials or travelers passing through. I am sure that you can stay there."

We traveled together a little farther before he turned and rode off into the farmlands. With the coolness of evening I received renewed strength and covered the miles in short order. At the entrance to Mahoba the police said to go through the village to the third road and turn left. As I turned down the third road, it was getting darker. Soon I came to some dark woods. An old man came toward me, grinning from ear to ear. He had some teeth missing and a sprig of hair tied on the top of his head. Behind him stood a one-story building with a veranda.

"Oh, what am I getting into out in these deep woods?" I said out loud.

The sun was down, and as I stepped on the porch the rain increased. The little man seemed to be expecting me, and we hit it off immediately. Soon he was squatting on the floor in front of a little stove on which he boiled some water. He brought a pail of cold water for my bath. There was a bathroom with a cement floor, a squat-down toilet, and running water (the kind you run out to the well and bring in). Guests slept in their clothes, so the bed covers are not changed very often, and no curtains cluttered the view out the windows. But I felt as if I were in a palace. The cold bath refreshed my tired body, and soon I felt stronger and able to eat something. No more horns, no more curious onlookers—just somewhere to rest my exhausted body for the night. In spite of the difficulties, I'd covered 36 miles that day. Before going to sleep I said a prayer of gratitude for the miracles performed in my behalf. God had sent the young man out on the road at just the right time to tell me where I should go.

The next morning I continued to ride toward Sitapur. I arrived at the Mayur Hotel, across from the army base, about 10:00. The vines and flowers in the garden and the shade from the trees made it a restful place in the midst of the hustling throng. The proprietor, N. F. Zaida, spoke English well. I learned that he ran three businesses in the city.

I had covered only 25 miles, but for some reason I felt I should stay there until the next day. I asked Mr. Zaida if I might go to the kitchen and have the cook boil me some vegetables. (I didn't want them swimming in oil.) The cooks were making chapati on a block on the floor and preparing other foods with an unbelievable lack of sanitation. Of course, flies were everywhere, but this was a way of life and nobody thinks anything of it.

Several officials came by about 4:30. I met Dr. R. K. Tandon, a cardiologist who belonged to the Lions Club and encouraged me to stay for their meeting that evening. A reporter came to interview me and take pictures for the newspaper. Dr. Tandon offered to place a long-distance call to Gene, but we couldn't complete the call.

I went to the village in a rickshaw and shopped, unsuccessfully, for a pair of long pants that would be cool and not baggy. As I headed back to the hotel, herds of cows wandered aimlessly in the streets, where they had free run. It was very important for drivers to watch for the cows and not injure any of them. The Hindus didn't believe in killing any living thing. I felt sorry for the cows. Some of them were eating paper, just to get something in their stomachs. The pitiful garbage left by hungry humans and filthy water in the puddles provided their daily fare.

The Lions Club met at 10:00 p.m. Some of the wives came, dressed in beautiful saris. Everyone made me feel very much at home. I spoke about the benefits of making health a high priority in our lives, and how men and women in the business and professional fields seem to get less exercise and become less physically fit as time goes on. They invited me to join them for dinner after the meeting. Since I had eaten earlier and knew I had to get up at 5:30 in the morning, I declined their invitation.

My room had curtainless windows in the door and large windows facing out to the passageway where people walked by. The Indian people sleep clothed and without covers, so I guess it doesn't matter if the world passes by while you are asleep. Nevertheless, I taped some newspapers up to afford myself a little more privacy.

The next morning high spirits were the order of the day. I headed east with the wind at my back and three bottles of boiled water aboard my bike. But twenty-five miles down the road I didn't feel like singing so loud. I stopped to rest under a willow tree and enjoy a banquet of whole-wheat toast, oranges, and a boiled egg. That afternoon I pushed my bike for a while on the side of the road that had shade. By 3:00 my water bottles were almost empty.

They make a good-tasting mango juice drink in India, although not under the most sanitary conditions. I bought some from a vendor, but after two bottles I was more thirsty than ever from the sugar.

I reached Lucknow at 5:00 and got a real shock. I felt as if I were trying to ride through New York City on a bicycle. I maneuvered through two or three miles of bikes, cars, and animals pulling carts before I located the school where I would stay. The traffic was so close that my left handlebar caught a man's shirt sleeve, and I was thrown from my bike. Fortunately, the fall didn't hurt me.

I finally reached the school, and a Mr. and Mrs. James met me inside the compound and invited me to stay with them. I was so thirsty it was difficult to wait until some water boiled and cooled a little before I drank it. No matter how much I drank I couldn't quench my thirst. After a cold bath, drawn from a wall tap that drained onto the cement floor, I enjoyed a good night's sleep. I had covered 54 miles that day.

The next day we went into the heart of the city and visited an ancient British stronghold that had been devastated by a Muslim holy war. Five hundred people trapped in the bowels of the building had died of starvation. That evening Mr. and Mrs. James rode on his motorbike to accompany me the three miles to the train station in Lucknow, where I would catch a train to Varanasi. As we sat on the platform to watch for the train, I looked at the people around me and wondered which was worse—dying from too little to eat, or dying from cancer, coronaries, strokes, or diabetes caused by an overabundance of refined foods. I wished life could be the middle road for all people of the world.

CHASED AT HIGH NOON

The train ride to Varanasi was a delight compared to my first experience on the train in Pakistan. This air-conditioned train had comfortable beds, furnished with white linens. I was the only woman in a compartment with three men, and everybody just slept in their clothes. When I got off the train, I experienced a moment of anxiety until I located my bike. Then I needed to find an airline office and a place to eat my breakfast. The porters argued over who would assist me with my bike and take me where I wanted to go. One fellow knew just where to go and declared there would be no charge. But once we arrived at the hotel, my self-appointed guide asked for 10 rupees, a good sum for his services.

The proprietor of the hotel spoke English and was very kind. He even let me eat my breakfast seated on the couch in front of his office. It was Sunday, and the airline office wouldn't open until afternoon. *There must be some way to make connections to Katmandu,* I thought.

There was. A man in a white suit told me, "You can get on Air India to Katmandu. A taxi will take you to the airport for 70 rupees."

No, he wasn't an angel—just a ticket agent. But I appreciated his help. I got everything taken care of (including the bike), made it through customs, and by 10:45 was on my way again. While waiting to board the plane, I met a young woman named Sarah Scott. After landing, Sarah and I decided to stay at a hotel suggested by a man on the shuttle bus. He rode the bus specifically to invite people to this particular hotel. The price was right: We paid only $5 for the two of us.

Sarah, short, with long, blond hair, knew how to rough it and didn't mind the most primitive living conditions. Like many other girls, she was traveling alone to see the world before settling down. She proved to be a wonderful companion for several days in Nepal. We wandered around the square looking into the shops. I bought some German whole-wheat bread, and we each had a piece of apple pie. It didn't taste like pie back home, but it filled the hollow space inside. Sarah was a little under the weather that night, but we were happy to be inside, clean, and with a place to sleep.

The next day we walked at least five miles around the city. Entrepreneurs had started restaurants where the food and water were safe for the droves of foreigners visiting the city. Except for the rickshaws and dirt streets, we could have been walking down a street in New York. We stopped at the post office to see if anyone had sent us mail. I would have been overjoyed to find a letter from home, but hadn't planned a mail drop here. We took a rickshaw back to the Valley View Hotel, where we decided to share a room for one more night.

The next day I left my things in the hotel office and my bike in a safe place while I helped Sarah get settled on the fourth floor of her hostel. Then we walked out to a mission run by a group from Australia that gave shelter to hurt or sick foreigners. When we got back to town, I decided to move to Sarah's hostel. It cost only $2 or $3 a night. Steep, winding stairs led down to the bathroom three or four floors below.

We decided we'd try to get a glimpse of the famous Mount Everest and surrounding peaks. Some people saw the glory of it all, but because of the cloud cover others returned home without even a glimpse of the mountain. Sarah rented a bicycle and we started out on Wednesday, May 4, to climb into the foothills.

We passed small villages along the tree-lined roadside. Out in the country when rain began to fall we used hand motions to ask permission to wait out the downpour under the porch of a nearby house. The people had few earthly possessions. Someone was carding wool, sitting on the dirt floor. A grandma came from the fields with a bundle of grain stalks. The rain stopped after a half hour and we resumed our trip. Several children followed us for about a mile, but left us at the top of the next hill.

We decided to stop at Sheen Memorial Hospital. The road to the hospital was so steep that I couldn't climb up and push my loaded bike at the same time. So I left the cycle on its side and climbed the rest of the way to the top and asked someone to help me get my bicycle up the mountainside.

Once at the hospital, I felt a twinge of pride to be part of this army of medical personnel encompassing the globe. We met the medical director, N. E. Hein, M.D., from Argentina, and some of the other staff members. Everyone was busy, for this was the only place for miles around where the sick could come for care. I wondered how they could possibly give good care (by U.S. standards) with what they had to work with.

Both Sarah and I had diarrhea. The lab technician took stool cultures and both came back negative. The doctor gave me some medication to ease things a little. That night we stayed in the guest house and fixed our own meal, using the food we'd brought and some vegetables the staff members' wives gave us. During the night the mosquitoes attacked us. I decided to ignore them, but Sarah couldn't sleep and was up and down all night killing them.

The next day we climbed to a vantage point from which we could look out across the foothills and get a panoramic view of the highest mountain chain in the world. It was too hazy to see Mount Everest, but we were able to see several other mountains quite clearly. These mountains take one's breath away.

We left back at 11:00 and coasted much of the way, stopping at the village of Bhaktapur to eat lunch. The flies were so thick it was impossible to keep them away. We arrived in Katmandu by 5:00, which gave me time to buy some food and find the home of Paul and Dawn Dulhunty and their children. The Dulhuntys work for the Adventist Development and Relief Agency (ADRA), a humanitarian agency that sends dedicated workers all over the world to help in development and disaster relief. In Nepal, the Dulhuntys have vastly improved the living conditions for lepers and other unfortunate persons. What a delight to be in their clean, well-managed home, off the busy street, and able to understand the language! While Sarah went back to her hostel, I welcomed the opportunity to stay on the compound and take care of some cleaning chores.

The next morning we loaded into the Land Rover to attend church. After the service we stopped beside a river to enjoy our picnic lunch, and for a few hours we forgot the problems we would each be dealing with in the coming week. On the way home Paul picked up two leper patients, who had been in the hospital for treatment, to give them a ride to the leper colony.

In all my years, I'd never seen anything called a road that compared with the one into the colony. Deep holes, washouts, unbelievable ups and downs—yet Paul drove along as if he were simply out for an afternoon drive. Conditions at the leper colony told a story of dedication and love. Two years before, the people had been angry and dangerous, cast out from society. Paul and his team had helped change their lives drastically. Now everything was clean and orderly in the building where they lived. Though they didn't always have enough nourishing food, their situation was still a wonderful change from what they had known before. About 2,000 lepers live at the colony, 500 of whom are active cases. Many of them threw their arms around us in greeting.

Because time was slipping away I decided to head for Pokhara, east of Katmandu, then leave for Thailand when I returned. Dawn took me to the travel agency to purchase tickets to Calcutta and on to Bangkok. There seemed to be some trouble stirring between India and Bangladesh. The border between the two countries had closed while I was in Nepal. Cholera had broken out in Dhaka.

Dawn rode her bike alongside mine the next morning to see me safely out of town. We left before 7:00 and the traffic was light. After she turned around and started back, that now-familiar feeling of being alone in a strange land swept over me. For the next two hours the road climbed upward, then I hit a long downhill stretch. The monsoons had gutted the road in some places, and I worried that my brakes might burn out because I had to brake so much of the way down the hill. I rode through rolling hills with their constant up-down-up-down. The temperature climbed to 110°F., and the sun was directly overhead. I needed to find a shady place to rest. Usually I have energy to spare, but out there I knew the sun would kill me if I didn't escape its fury. My eyes burned and my throat was dry.

I ate lunch under a tree, then lay down to rest. A large, dark brown dog came and sat down near me, staying until I got up to leave after my nap. Two hours later I leaned against a rock under a shade tree and decided to write in my journal while I rested. A little boy came and sat down beside me. Although he stayed for more than an hour, we never exchanged a word.

Because of the heat and the hills I didn't make it to Mugu, the halfway point between Katmandu and Pokhara. Instead, I stopped in the little village of Gandak, which is little more than a wide space in the road. The village boasted two restaurants, a truck stop, and bathroom facilities on the ground in the woods. The truck stop would provide a roof over my head for the night. The young attendant offered me what was probably his own cot on the second floor. I asked him to boil some water for me.

I recognized the symptoms of heat exhaustion: fast, irregular pulse; air hunger; and prostration. My body needed help immediately. I lay on the cot, panting, trying to eat a whole-wheat bun and drink some pineapple juice. I knew my life was in the attendant's and God's hands. The attendant knelt down beside the little cot as I took in deep gulps of hot air. His tired eyes were full of compassion and understanding. He promised to help me the best way he knew how. After an hour I felt almost normal.

"Your bath is ready," my host announced with gestures and a few English words. "Please come with me."

He had placed a large kettle filled with water out in the front courtyard. I noticed an audience was already gathering. Women in India and Nepal take their baths at the water's edge or beside the village pump, washing with their soiled sari still on. At the end of the bath they do a magic exchange for a dry sari.

"How can I take a bath out here, Singh?" I asked.

So he picked up the heavy kettle and carried it to the lean-to attached to the building. There I had the privacy I needed for my bath. I soaped down, then stood in the kettle, pouring the cool water over my hot body. Suddenly I stopped. What was that in the bottom of the kettle? It wasn't moving, so it couldn't be alive. Poking it with my finger, I discovered it was my watch that had fallen from my shorts pocket.

Back in my little room I could hear dogs barking and trucks roaring their motors on the street. Through the wide gaps in the boards between the rooms it was possible to see and hear truckers coming and going all during the night. When I left the next morning, Singh looked red-eyed and exhausted. He'd been disturbed frequently during the night to accommodate the truckers. He filled my drinking bottles with boiled water, and I gave him seven rupees and waved goodbye, wishing something could be done to lighten his load.

As I rode out of Gandak I looked at the foothills across the valley. I watched farm families as they worked the earth and felt more secure with them close by as I walked and rode along.

Then just ahead were two bushy-haired men. They don't look like the Nepalese farmers. Their feet were bare, and they wore wraparound skirts that came above their knees. They walked, one on each side of the road, holding two bamboo poles stretched across the road between them. I couldn't ride under their barricade. I looked around, suddenly realizing I had climbed above the farmlands and was alone on the road. Only 100 feet remained between the men and me.

Did they belong to a bandit gang?

The men hadn't heard me coming. That part of the road was paved, and I knew I would be going downhill as soon as I got on the other side of their barricade. I was only 10 feet behind them now, and still neither of them turned around. Just as I reached the fellow on the left, I put my thumb on my bicycle bell and let it ring out shrilly across the still air. Startled, the man threw up his pole and jumped high in the air. I rushed through the open space. Seconds later, a wild, angry shout rang across the valley. I glanced over my shoulder and saw one of the men running toward me. He was only 15 feet away and running like a deer in his bare feet. He was so close and coming so fast that escape didn't seem possible. I shifted the bike into the lowest gear and set a new world record for all senior citizens as I sped away from my pursuer. I didn't look back until I began to climb the next hill beyond a turn in the road. By then my pursuers were small figures on the road above. The terrifying memory of the bandit's angry shout returned to frighten me long after the danger had passed.

I hurried to the village of Mugu, a mile or so away. My watch said it was 5:00. (It had gained four hours, but I didn't know that. The water bath hadn't done it any good.) I decided to leave my bike with the police in Mugu, ride the bus to Pokhara to see Annapurna Himal, then return to Mugu and pick up my bike and ride the bus back to Katmandu. From Katmandu I would fly to Calcutta and Bangkok before riding toward Singapore.

I had time to eat and find a safe place to leave my bike before the bus came through at 3:00. On the bus, many people were standing, and some had chickens or other strange baggage, but everyone seemed to accept the crowded conditions. As the driver gunned the motor to get past the washed out areas on the curving roads, the passengers were thrown to the left, and then to the right, as if everyone were doing a strange square dance.

We arrived in Pokhara just before sundown and I found a hotel. As I drifted off to sleep, I gave thanks for making it safely through the day. I was thankful that the bus driver had made it around those treacherous curves. I also realized that if my watch hadn't gained four hours, it was possible I would have gone on past Mugu, thinking I had plenty of time before dark. Most of all, what would have happened if I hadn't gotten away from the pursuing mountain man?

When I went up to the rooftop the next day the whole Annapurna mountain chain was visible. Incredible! I had my watch repaired at a watchmaker's shop in the village, then enjoyed dinner with other travelers. Afterward I walked down to the lake. Children went to the bathroom on the bank of the lake, women washed their clothes in the lake, and still others swam in the lake. Even so, I wondered if the lake was any more contaminated than the streams and rivers at home.

Fortunately I managed to get the bus back to Katmandu. On my way to Dawn and Paul's house, I passed the U.S. Embassy and stopped to talk to the Nepalese guard at the gate about the men with the bamboo poles. With tears in his eyes, he said, "Thank God you got away!"

Dawn helped me do my laundry. Then that evening eight student missionaries came over for singing and refreshments. On the way to Sheen Hospital with the Dulhunty family for church services the next morning, we rode over shocks of wheat laid in the road. The tires of trucks and cars thrashed the wheat as they drove across. The terraced hills and red soil blended with the blue sky to paint a canvas only God could make. That evening the Dulhuntys and Dez Thompson, a teacher for the lepers, took me to supper at one of the large hotels. They said this weekly respite helped them get through some of the almost intolerable situations during the week.

The next morning I awoke early to have time to listen to some tapes on the life of Christ and to pray for guidance and protection on the journey ahead of me. I needed to keep the channels open so that I would be aware of His voice and not choose my own way. I caught up on my journal, finished my news report, and was ready to head to the airport. My next stop would be Calcutta.

I got a hotel room in a village near Calcutta. The air conditioner clanged and rattled in its efforts to cool the air. After a brief rest, I decided to visit some places of interest in the city. I hired a taxi to drive me around and covered a lot of ground. I stopped at the Missionaries of Poverty. Mother Teresa was in France at the time, so I missed seeing her. Their mission is very clean and the people well cared for. I saw mostly children there.

Our next stop was the Ganges River that people use for anything and everything. The destitute live under trees or in makeshift boxes not far from its banks. I stopped along the roadside and talked with a group of lepers. I gave a man a little money for food for his wife, but what would he do tomorrow? I bought some water, film, and fruit before heading back to the hotel. Tomorrow I would wing my way toward a new land.

HIT FROM BEHIND IN THAILAND

Mrs. Audrey Wilcox, the Thailand Mission president's secretary, picked me up at the Thai airport, and I stayed at her home during my visit. I spoke in worship the next morning. My message never varied greatly, for what I was doing told a story of its own. I hoped that some of the people who heard me speak would consider a change in their own lifestyle. Most of us in some way, whether through too much work, too much stress, or too little exercise, cut short our stay here on earth.

I took my bike to a bike shop to repair a bent sprocket and get a general check for loose nuts and bolts. When I was ready to leave, Audrey took me to the outskirts of the city, and once more I was on a road in a foreign land, wondering what the day would bring. It rained that morning, and I stopped under a shelter until the storm passed. Back on the road once more, it was not long until I came to a place where water covered the road. I followed the cars through the muddy water. On and on we went. Luckily I was able to keep up with the slow-moving traffic and breathed a sigh of relief when I finally reached dry ground..

Traffic was more orderly here, with fewer exhaust fumes and no blowing horns. What a relief! The cars moved rapidly, however, and the shoulder was poor to nonexistent. Suddenly, *wham!* Something hit me. I was catapulted onto sharp rocks imbedded in the shoulder of the road, landing on my hands and knees. Blood flowed freely from a deep gouge in my left knee and several abrasions and lacerations. As soon as I got up and determined I could walk and had no broken bones, my attention went to my bicycle. The board that supported the right pannier in back was broken. Several men stopped and offered to take me in their car to see a doctor. I tried to explain that I must ride there. They probably thought I had hit my head. A policeman came by and determined from witnesses that I'd been hit by a motorcycle.

I finally followed the men to the doctor's office. The doctor bandaged me up and gave me some antibiotics. He said my wounds would take a long time to heal. I wanted to pay the bill, but apparently the man who hit me was responsible for the charges. If I thought I attracted attention before, it was nothing compared to the stares I got as I pedaled my bandaged body down the road. I did not really crave this extra windfall of attention.

I stopped for dinner at a little restaurant on the edge of town. My poor old knee felt better propped up on a chair. After I ate, I rested and did some writing. Sitting in a chair would not get me any farther south, though, so I started out once more.

In Samut Songkhram I stopped at a drugstore. The pharmacist and his wife spoke English and were most helpful. (While there I met a young man from Kalamazoo, Michigan, about an hour's drive from my home!) The pharmacist took me to the Alongkorn Neighbor Hotel. In spite of everything, I'd traveled 42 miles that day and looked forward to a good night's rest. There were no flies to get on my wounds, it was cool, and the price was only $6 for the night.

It took me half an hour to get out of town the next morning, because I shared the road with a very large Brahman bull and some cattle. When I stopped to eat, the water in my drinking bottle was hot enough to make mashed potatoes. Beans from a can, two peeled tomatoes, two small cucumbers, and whole-wheat bread completed my meal. The roadside cafe where I stopped allowed me to rest on a cot in back. In spite of the swarms of flies, unsanitary conditions, and sweat dripping from my body, I slept about an hour.

By 3:30 heat exhaustion overwhelmed me, so I stretched out on a bench in a grove of trees off the road. A young girl brought me some cold water, but I didn't dare drink it. I was gasping for breath and my pulse raced. I poured the cold water over myself to help cool my body. The girl invited me to come into the backyard where I rested on a bed and tried to eat some fruit and nuts. I enjoyed watching her rock her baby, talking softly and sweetly.

The girl's mother rode up on a motorbike. Her name was Lami Ansaard, and she said she taught in the village and could speak some English. They invited me to spend the night with them, which meant I didn't have to travel the 7.2 miles to get to Phetchabun, the next town. I traveled only 26.8 miles that day, but it was late and I needed to rest. The bathroom had facilities for taking a bath, which helped to refresh my spirits. It seemed I rallied fairly quickly once I got off the road.

There must be a way I can get out of this intense heat and humidity, I thought. I went into Phetchabun the next morning. I had to get into an air-conditioned hotel to replenish my energy and change my bandages. The cuts were healing nicely, but my knee was draining. At the hotel I put on fresh bandages, then took some food to a restaurant on the corner where they cooked it for me. The father, curious to know all about me, went through my folder of information about the trip. I enjoyed a visit with his family while I ate.

As I rode along the next day I saw a young couple in the distance coming toward me. We stopped along the road and chatted for a few minutes. Monica and David Murtach from Australia said they were cycling from England to Australia, covering 24 to 36 miles a day.

It was only 9:00, but already the heat began to take its toll on me. *I must rest more,* I thought. I poured water over myself to wet down my clothes, but they were dry again before I reached the next bend in the road. I stopped at a small eating place and bought some vegetables. I asked the woman if I could put my pot on the fire. In no time my vegetables and pan were burned beyond recognition. Well, my load had gotten a little lighter, if nothing else. I was without a stove, a kettle, a flashlight, and a meter, but my courage was still on top. An open sore on the calf of my leg refused to heal, so I tried to get some sun on it. But I had to keep it covered most of the time because of the flies.

In Cha-Am I paid more for a room than at any place in Asia. The first night it cost $8 for a room with a fan. The next night it cost $12 for a room with air-conditioning. I met a young couple there from Germany. Klaus and Verena Wagner were both physicians and suggested that I not put my body under so much stress from the heat.

"Why don't you go to China, where it is still a little cooler, and ride some extra miles there?"

I felt strongly impressed to follow their advice. I would take the train to Singapore, then fly to Hong Kong, or possibly go on to Australia, and return before going into China. I wanted to go under my own power to Hua Hin so that I would have a definite beginning and finishing city in Thailand.

I was on the road early before it got hot. A cloud covered the sun part of the time, and I rode on the shady side of the road whenever possible. I arrived in Hua Hin about 10:00 and went to the train station. The train would leave at 7:00 p.m. and arrive in Butterworth the next day. At the station I met a Japanese journalist, who was preparing an article for a Japanese journal, *Update*. She wanted to arrange an interview when I arrived in Tokyo. Food stalls I visited while I waited for the train offered a better selection than I had seen in other countries.

The train was wonderful—efficient and smooth running with clean, comfortable berths. As I rode along I sought guidance as to whether I should go to Australia. The cost to get there would be $700, and the rainy season had already begun. The cost, time, and rain were not in my favor. I would know what to do when I reached Singapore.

I enjoyed a wonderful and refreshing sleep on the train. My memory wandered back to Pakistan and the ride to Lahore in third-class. I will always be grateful for that experience! It made everything else seem first-class by comparison. My wounds continued to heal. Air conditioning and lack of flies and sweat helped the process considerably.

When I arrived in Butterworth, the second-class air-conditioned trains for Singapore were full. I couldn't take my bike on the next train, so I decided to wait until the next day. I went to Penang and rode a rickshaw around the city for 45 minutes. The city looked very prosperous, but I heard that drugs were rampant there.

I rode the train to Singapore the next day. A bus from the Seventh-day Adventist headquarters picked me up at the station. I was given a lovely apartment, and for the next few days felt as if I was home with family. I had the bike repaired and enjoyed the opportunity to meet with old friends and catch up on what they'd been doing. I also got to go shopping, but was disappointed when I couldn't find a Cateye meter. The night before I left for the trip into Hong Kong and China, I went to sleep, confident that God had helped me make the right choice.

CHINA, LAND OF WONDER

It was June 1. I was on my way to Hong Kong. When I arrived, I wasn't sure which mission compound to contact, so I called Connie Ash in the Health Education Department. We met at the Hyatt Hotel and took a taxi to Tsuen Wan Adventist Hospital, where she lived in an apartment.

Somehow I needed to find out what was expected of me as a cyclist in China. I called a bicycle shop that also managed bike tours. The manager's answers to my questions left me with a pretty grim outlook. According to him it was against the law to bring bikes into China. I would have to stay in expensive foreign hotels, I couldn't ride without going in a group, a meter would cost $210, and I would have to take my bike apart. Again I asked for God's guidance.

Then I met Phillip Wong. He was in Hong Kong to help renovate the hospital. He took me and my bike to a good cycle shop, and then took me back later to pick it up. He drove me a long way to a little shop where I found a Cateye meter for only $26!

When I went to the travel bureau to get my visa for China, I was told I wouldn't have to take my cycle apart and I could take it to China with me. I could pick up my visa the next day, and all I needed was one picture and $10. Thanks to the care and hospitality of many people, I managed to get everything ready for my trip into China.

A friend advised me to contact Mr. Wong Lee (not his real name) when I arrived in Beijing. I didn't have his phone number, however, and he lived in a city of several million people. Again, I needed help from above. I had just enough Hong Kong money to get a taxi to the airport, something for my stay, and airport registration. The people at the airport assisted me in every way, and I was soon on my way to the People's Republic of China. My assigned helper at the airport found the needed information on Mr. Lee before my flight left.

When I landed in Beijing, a young man from the foreign affairs office helped me phone Mr. Lee. Then the young man, who had come to the airport to pick up a guest, invited me to ride with them into Beijing. I took a taxi to the Beijing Hotel, where I was to meet Mr. Lee. He rode up to the hotel entrance on his bicycle. (Few Chinese have cars of their own.) I had my bike, but the front tire was flat, so we started to his house pushing our bikes. As we passed Tieneman Square, the flag was being lowered, and hundreds of cyclists and shoppers stopped and silently waited.

Bicycle lanes on either side of the highway often spilled out into the main traffic. Some commuters travel as much as two hours each way to work. We walked three miles to Mr. Lee's simple but comfortable home with a fenced-in courtyard in back. His wife prepared a nice supper for us. While we ate, his son, who lived on the property, took the tire off my bike and checked it. He couldn't find anything wrong with it. Once he pumped it up it seemed to be fine. I thanked them for their help and hospitality, then Mr. Lee and I left to find a hotel. Foreigners are supposed to stay in hotels built for them, but there are alternatives. We covered about 10 miles, pedaling in and out of the busy traffic as we looked for a hotel I felt I could afford.

"There is one more place," Mr. Lee said. "If we cannot get you in there my son will keep you overnight, even though it is against the law in China to keep a foreigner overnight. Because I am a teacher, I must not take the risk of disobeying the law." I could see the anxiety on his face as he spoke.

The last place we stopped was a very large hostel. After much discussion I learned a bed was available downstairs in a three-bed room that had a bathroom across the hall.

The next morning I was ready to tackle China. I headed for breakfast in the dining room and waited 45 minutes for my order to arrive. I had ordered two eggs, boiled for 10 minutes. What the waitress brought me was 10 boiled eggs piled high on a plate. All of us enjoyed a good laugh at the misunderstanding.

I decided against exchanging money on the black market, even though nearly everyone did it. A clear conscience was easier to live with, and I didn't want any problems as I traveled. It rained most of the day, so I spent my first full day in China catching up my journal entries.

One of my roommates at the hostel was Michelle, a young French woman. Michelle, her boyfriend Eugene, and I traveled all over the city on our bikes the next day. Eugene led the way, weaving in and out of traffic, while Michelle and I darted around things, trying not to run into anyone, but still keep up with Eugene.

There were so many things to see—the 30-meter-high temple of Buddha, gold and silver everywhere, and many rich carvings. To worship things made of wood and stone when there is a living Christ seemed strange to me, but maybe the things we spend our time, money, and effort on are just as useless, as far as bringing us happiness and peace of mind. We rode more than 17 miles on our bikes as we traveled from place to place. I was thankful to still be alive when we got back to the hostel.

The next day nine of us rode in a van to the Great Wall of China, a two-and-a-half-hour trip. The wall, like a long ribbon, stretches as far as one can see. The first section of the wall was finished in 221 B.C., requiring 300,000 men to complete it. Many lost their lives when enemies came from the north, bribed the gatekeeper, and marched right through the gate.

After our visit, the others planned to return on the bus, but I wanted to ride my bicycle back to Beijing. I knew I needed to start early to reach Beijing before dark—it would take a couple hours just to get across the city. It was downhill for a while, coming off the mountain, then turned into a slight, but steady, climb for miles. Wong Gong, a young student, accompanied me. He practiced his English on me for several miles. Then, somehow, the front wheel of my bicycle hit his front wheel. We were moving fairly fast, and the impact threw me over the back of his bike. I twisted my left leg so that it hurt to stand on it. Now there was another deep gouge in my left knee. Blood also oozed from my left hand, but fortunately I had not hit my head.

Wong helped me apply some bandages, and we started down the hill again. At first I seemed able to keep going, then things gradually got worse. I felt faint and was afraid I might fall off the bike. We reached the place where Wong should turn east toward his own home, but he stayed with me. Finally, I stopped. I couldn't go any farther. I could hardly walk, and sat down at a table. Wong tried to flag down a car to take me into Beijing. Finally, two young executive types stopped. They put my bike in the trunk of the car and helped me into the back seat. By the time we found the hostel I couldn't walk, so one of them carried me down to my room and put me on the bed.

My roommate in the next bed, a girl from London, was a physician. "No bones are broken," she told me, "but you aren't going anywhere, Charlotte, until that leg heals. The wounds will heal easier than the leg."

I knew she was right. I must rest so that the damaged muscles could heal properly. Right then, I was glad to be in bed, catching my breath. I was also thankful that the bathroom was so close to our bedroom, although earlier I had complained about the smell. For several days I hobbled along, not able to walk very well, managing only to get to the dining room and small store on the hostel grounds. My roommates brought me things I needed and let me take their arms to steady my shuffling steps. Even the desk helpers softened a little and let me lean on them. I put heat on my wounds and they scabbed over quickly, but had little volcanoes erupting underneath.

My leg felt so much better by Tuesday that I went to the lobby looking for someone to share a taxi with me. A tour leader from Poland invited me to join her group. Eleven of us rode the mini-bus and visited Friendship Market, set up especially for foreigners, stocked with canned and bakery goods, juice, brown bread, and raisin rolls, among other things. I had some film developed, then labeled the pictures, and mailed them home. After all that, guess who spent most of the next day in bed!

I had a decision that required earnest prayer. Greg, a young American, wanted to accompany me. He thought the excitement of riding into the interior of China as a guide was something he would like to tackle. There was something about him that seemed right, and I went with him to the U.S. Embassy to see if he could get his visa extended. The gentleman at the counter was adamant.

"You have already extended your stay twice. Now be out of China in 11 days!"

On Monday, June 20, I asked God to help me be back on the road by Wednesday. I knew the leg injury was not that much better, but I trusted in some special help, should it be necessary. I took a taxi to the security bureau to extend my visa for another month.

The next morning it still hurt as much as ever to walk on my leg. That afternoon I spoke to the nurses at the Chou Yong Hospital, where Hong Rong Guan, a medical doctor, was doing his graduate work. He also wanted to accompany me to the interior. I spoke through an interpreter to about 200 nurses attending the meeting. Afterward, they presented me with a medallion of the hospital and a bamboo picture. I had taken two low potency Motrin at 1:00, and realized during the afternoon that I was keeping up with the others as we walked around the hospital. At midnight I still had no pain. Perhaps the pills had eased the pain enough to relax the injured muscles. I would like to feel that God was honoring my faith and answering my request to leave on Wednesday.

Wednesday morning I was up at 6:45 a.m. to finish packing. The leg felt fine. This was the biggest miracle yet! I took two more

Motrin. I'm not a pill taker, but with the miles of road I needed to cover before nightfall I felt there would be less stress on the leg if I took the Motrin.

For two weeks young Hong Rong had been asking to be my guide into the interior. Not sure about the legal implications should he get hurt, I hesitated. But since Greg had to leave, I decided to let Hong Rong Guan accompany me. We headed south over the Yellow River and east toward the Pacific Ocean. Bicycle traffic was heavy on the highway. With Guan leading the way, we moved along at about nine miles per hour. Once we were in the country the traffic thinned out. The roads were good and my leg felt fine. Guan did well with his one-speed. He might have had some sore muscles, but he didn't admit it. We had gone 45 miles by 5:30, in spite of a strong head wind. We stopped at a hostel overnight. By U.S. standards the place would be considered primitive, but the best thing was that wherever we stopped, the Chinese always had large thermoses of hot water they used for making tea. So I didn't have to stop and boil water for drinking. We cooked our meals on Guan's little stove that used liquid fuel in a cup.

By Friday we had reached Changzhou. My front tire had been slowly going flat. At a roadside bike shop the owner told us the tube was not only bent inside the tire, but was also too long and had been put in wrong. He fixed the tire and I had no further trouble with it. In the afternoon Guan's bicycle had a flat tire. I decided to pedal on, as it was necessary for me to ride from point A to point B under my own power. Guan caught a ride on a tractor and would catch up with me after he got his tire fixed.

I rode by vegetable gardens and orchards. Sometimes trees lined both sides of the road, which made the air a little cooler. Some of the peasants I met had everything imaginable loaded on their bicycles. I was making pretty good time, riding along on a good shoulder, my head down, and my mind obviously not where it belonged. I suddenly slammed into the back of a heavy truck. My cycle flew under the truck and hit the wheel. The impact threw me to the ground. I thank God my head was down when I hit forehead first. The impact split the back of my helmet. My face could have been mashed otherwise!

Three men jumped out and raced to the back of the truck, staring at me in silence. They wanted to lift me up, but I motioned for them to wait. I needed to catch my breath and absorb the shock. When I did stand up, my head ached for about 30 seconds, then the ache disappeared. How do you straighten out such an incident when you can't speak each other's language? A bicycle running into a stopped truck is a very unusual thing. I started to laugh, and soon we were all laughing. The bicycle survived the crash just fine, and after a while Guan arrived and we were on our way again.

I made 30 more miles that day, added to 30 miles already behind me before I hit the truck. We ended up at a fancy hotel in Tsangchow, where we received a royal welcome. On Sabbath morning we enjoyed a tasty Chinese breakfast in our honor. I was getting a little skinny and didn't want to start burning muscle for fuel. My leg started to hurt while we were walking that afternoon. After I rested a while the pain disappeared. That was the last of the real pain, and it never came back again.

A strong head wind the next day kept us from doing more than six miles per hour when we rode on a slight grade. In spite of the wind we covered 55 miles.

My unhealed wounds concerned Guan. He soaked my nail scissors in boiling water, cut off the dead skin, then cleaned the sores. He crushed a couple of the antibiotic tablets I had with me and filled the knee cavity and the sore on my calf. The next night he did it again. He also wanted me to take antibiotics by mouth for at least a couple days. After that the wounds healed nicely.

On Monday we stopped at an oil company hotel to see what it would cost to stay there. A policeman showed up and asked me for some identification. I didn't have a bike permit, which was issued mainly for tours and for riding in restricted areas.

Guan presented my case. "In America, travelers can go anywhere. We are just riding along this road. Mrs. Hamlin is not interested in our security facilities. She loves the Chinese people and everywhere is encouraging people to live a healthy lifestyle so they'll be able to do more for themselves when they get older."

God was on our side. I was given a hotel room with a private bath. Guan shared a room down the hall. The next day Guan said, "From now on, we'll stay in the hostels and dirt. There's less red tape and fuss." That was fine with me.

My meter registered only 46.32 miles. We needed to move along faster. We crossed the famous Yellow River and headed into hilly country. Open spaces with farm land and little homes dotted the countryside. Every time we stopped to rest, people asked who I was, why I was dressed so differently, and where I was going. Sometimes Guan would translate a short talk to the people gathered around.

Near Tsinan was the High Mountain. Hikers considered it a great honor to climb to the top and watch the sunrise. Guan made the trip on his bicycle without me, leaving about 10:00 p.m. and returning the next morning. He slept an hour, then we were on our way again.

That evening we rode for two hours after dark, which was very dangerous. When we finally came to a motel-like building, we were happy to get off the road for the night. They charged us twice as much as usual, which upset Guan, but I told him to calm down. Had we continued riding in the dark we might not have made it at all.

One day I decided to go from the bicycle lane, which had very "wavy" pavement, onto the side of the freeway. I didn't take time to glance in the rearview mirror first and collided with a man coming up behind me. I went down on my left knee (of course) and the bicycle landed on top of me. The poor man became very excited and tried to lift me to my feet. I did my best to ask him to first remove the bike from on top of me. When I was back on my feet, I asked him if he was all right. He nodded that all was well, I touched him on the shoulder, and we both laughed.

I had not seen another White face since I left Beijing. Other cyclists rode along behind me and watched as I changed gears, which were quite a novelty to them. When we sat down for lunch in a little restaurant, so many people crowded around us that Guan thought he would suffocate, though I really felt he enjoyed himself and all the attention. In the early afternoon I noticed sealant oozing out of the front tire, the result of a fence nail embedded in the tire. We decided to fix it right there with a little kit I had in my bag.

"Let's go over there by that little business and get in the shade first," Guan suggested.

The sign said Coal for Sale, but it was also a bicycle shop. The man fixed the tire, but before I rode very far it was flat again. I decided it was time to put on both a new tire and a new tube, which I had with me. I had not had one blowout since I left Belgium, crossed Europe, and got this far into Asia.

DETAINED IN FORBIDDEN TERRITORY

Since a week had passed since our last rest day, we stopped at a hotel. I looked down from the third floor to the courtyard below, where customers were being served. A customer took his bowl of bean soup, then went to the bread table and took what he wanted. When he brought the bowl back, it was rinsed in a container and was ready for the next customer.

A couple police officers came to see us. Guan explained the purpose of our trip and where we were going. The policemen left, and we considered the matter closed. Guan had suggested earlier that I exchange money on the black market so we would have more money for our expenses. "If you will be patient," I told him, "my honesty will pay off in the end."

The next morning the police wanted to see us again. When they talked to Guan for an hour, he became very worried. Tourists were running here and there without permits but usually weren't confronted, it seems, unless something unusual came up. They asked us to appear in a large room on the second floor. We sat down next to an official. A policeman sat to our left and a solemn figure stood across from us. Another policeman to my right wrote down everything. We were literally on the red carpet.

"You have disobeyed the law in China," said the high district official. "You must be punished, and we must take your bicycle."

"That means that my tour is over, doesn't it?" I said.

"No, but why are you in China?" he asked.

"I am here on a good will tour for health."

"Do you have a bicycle permit to be out here on the road?"

"No," I admitted. "It is my fault that I don't have one with me. For that I cannot blame the Chinese government."

"Do you know that you are in forbidden territory here in China?"

"We are traveling on the freeway toward Shanghai, where I will be going by plane to Japan. The Chinese people have been very good to me on the way."

Guan told them that I was honest and would not even exchange money on the black market. He assured them I had no interest in visiting the army installation or other security areas. I had to sign a paper verifying what had been said. Then they told us to go upstairs. They would call me when they had made a decision. I asked Guan to kneel down with me and pray that God would intervene on our behalf. It may have been the first time he had ever listened to a plea to the living God.

Guan could be sentenced to 10 years in prison for being with me. As for me, they could take my bike to customs, fine me 100Y, give me a citation for breaking the law and being in forbidden territory, or put me in jail for 10 days, which would leave me with a criminal record.

They called us back to the room at 3:00 p.m. "Because you have not blamed the Chinese for what happened and admit that you yourself were responsible for not having a permit, and because you have come on a good will mission and would not exchange money on the black market, all charges are being dropped. But you must go on to Shanghai and finish riding there."

Two officers accompanied us to the bus station. We would take a bus to Tai'an and then a train to Shanghai. A staring crowd gathered in the waiting room, which annoyed the officers. We waved to the policemen as they left and felt we had parted as friends. I was thankful for the opportunity to get a glimpse into China as it really is and to meet people who were unchanged by the Western world. I regretted that Guan had to be tested along with me, though. It was a memorable experience for both of us.

We got a train almost immediately that night, and were in Shanghai the next morning. The date was July 4. After a restful sleep, we headed out of Shanghai city to visit the foreign student dormitory at Chinese University where the students came from many different countries. We talked to several of them. It can be a rewarding experience to discover that we don't have everything back home, and that there are many things we can learn outside our domain that are practical and add satisfaction and challenge to life.

The traffic was unbelievable! Guan remarked, "If my father knew I was riding a bicycle in Shanghai he would greatly disapprove."

We found the Bureau of Foreign Security. As we suspected, they wouldn't issue a permit to ride a bike outside the city of Shanghai. The penalty would be severe if Guan rode with me outside the allowed territory. In the evening we went back to the hostel, having traveled 20 hard-earned miles in Shanghai.

We were off again the next day to find a route through Shanghai that would get us to the airport. Even with signs everywhere, Guan had to inquire a number of times about the location of the airport. We dodged bicycles, taxis, pedestrians, and buses, but finally did arrive safely at the airport. I checked at China International Airlines about the bicycle. They would take it to Osaka, Japan.

Outside once more, we explored the area and found that we could ride around in sort of a circle on a lightly-traveled area. I told Guan to make sure we did not get into Forbidden Territory. We got back to the hostel at 8:00 with 12 hours and 47 miles to our credit. After getting myself and all my clothes cleaned and repacked (even my AROUND THE WORLD banner), I crawled into bed in a dormitory where many other foreigners were staying. Tomorrow I would arrive in the Land of the Rising Sun.

But I needed a way to the airport with my bicycle and luggage. Early the next morning I went across the street to the Shanghai Hotel to ask if a limousine might be going to the airport. No. There was nothing to do except go back, get my things ready, and keep praying. I must not miss that plane.

For some reason, I felt I should go back to the hotel again.

Parked right in front of the hotel door stood a shiny van. The driver was waiting to take two Japanese businessmen to the airport. I asked him if it might be possible for me to go along. My bike fit just right beside the middle seat, and the two businessmen sat in the back seats.

Guan came to tell me goodbye. I told him again how much I appreciated all he had done to help me and gave him money to help with his expenses on the trip home. He couldn't have helped but notice that I, a Christian, had been protected and cared for by a power stronger than any earthly power.

At the airport I breezed through the preliminaries without a hitch. A lawyer and his wife sat next to me while we waited to board the plane. He told me that from childhood the Chinese are taught "what is Chinese truth," and when difficulty arises they seem unable to reason and are helpless in finding a solution to the problem. He added, "But there is a harmony in their closeness to nature that helps them to cope, perhaps even better than we do."

DANGEROUS TUNNELS IN JAPAN

After two hours flight time we landed on the runway in Osaka, Japan. Pastor Inu from the Kōbe Adventist Hospital came to meet me. I was given a lovely guest room with a private bath and served delicious food. Everything was shiny and spotless. I could even drink water from the tap!

More than 30 years before I had started a Bible-English school in Kōbe. My husband had raised money in Japan to build the Osaka Center, not far from where I was staying. Things had changed over the years, though, and none of it seemed familiar.

The people at the hospital invited me out for dinner and supper and showed me every possible kindness. Chaplain Yasui asked me to speak to the boys and girls in the Pathfinder club on Sunday morning. As always, the children couldn't believe this grandma could possibly ride and ride and ride.

The *Asa Hi* newspaper, with a circulation of 800,000, sent a reporter to interview me. His picture of me with the Pathfinders appeared in the paper the next day over a short article about my trip. Although the Japanese have less cancer and fewer heart attacks, hypertension is fairly common. Hopefully, our interview might have had an impact on the journalist, the children, or some of the people who read the newspaper.

Pastor Yasui offered to take me to Kyōto as starting on the highway from Kōbe could be difficult. What a relief! I should have known all along that God had taken care of everything. We left in the afternoon and went to the Kyōto church that had a nice guest room in the back. Pastor Ebihara invited me to have supper with his family.

Tomorrow I would be on my own again, a stranger in a foreign land. Would I remember enough Japanese to make myself understood? I asked my heavenly Father to come along with me as I once more faced the unknown.

After breakfast Pastor Ebihara took me out to heavily traveled Highway One, a main route running north toward Tokyo. He changed my mirror over to the right side as, of course, I must ride to the left of cars here. We prayed together beside the road, then I was on my way.

The "1" is always on a large blue board which makes the route easy to spot. I moved along the narrow shoulder, sneaking to the front of the pack to wait for the light to change, then moving across before the semis and other vehicles could get into gear. After five hours in bumper-to-bumper traffic as one village ran into the next, I was ready to call it a day.

I stopped at a Chevron station to ask the owner if he knew of an inexpensive place I could stay. He called several places without success before he found a hostel. Thankfully, he took me over there, for I don't think I would have found it on my own. The room had four bunk beds and sliding doors leading to the courtyard. Men and women used the same bathroom. The bath was at the other end of the building, so I could have a wonderful soak in a hot tub. I needed it.

I was out by 7:00 the next morning, looking for my number "1" highway. The shoulder had disappeared, the sidewalks were rough, and it was hard to increase my speed. I prayed that I'd stay relaxed, for I knew it was hard on the system to stay tense hour after hour. Even though I didn't see other foreigners, people didn't stop and stare. Every day was a new experience. Sometimes I ate in restaurants; sometimes a family invited me to join them for a meal. As long as I asked for a Japanese inn, my search for lodging was over.

On the way to Fukaya I encountered many hills and heavy traffic. The bike trails were better, and sometimes the paths curved around by the sea. Somewhere along the way my highway turned into a fast moving freeway. Unfortunately, I was not allowed to stay on it. Riding through the hilly villages slowed my progress, and the chain on my bicycle broke while changing gears on a steep hill. That brought me to a halt until I could get it fixed. I walked along the road until I spotted a small business. It turned out to be a place for eye care needs. The optometrist's son straightened my glasses, and I bought a new pair of sunglasses. Then the father drove me in his pickup truck to a bicycle repair shop. The mechanic removed one link and rejoined the chain. Soon I was on my way again. People are so precious everywhere!

One afternoon I traveled through eight tunnels as I rode in the mountains. There were no bike trails, and I have a strong suspicion that bikes were not allowed in the tunnels. The semis and trucks barreled through like lightning. Pushing my bike, I walked along a narrow ledge against the tunnel wall like a person on a tight rope. One tunnel must have been a mile long.

One evening I stayed in a lovely little inn. My small table held a cake and some juice, a toothbrush, and tiny tube of toothpaste. The bathroom floors were of highly polished stone molded right into the flooring. Slippers worn in the toilet area were not worn out on the other floors. An inside garden had a fish pond, trees, flowers, and decorative stones. The whole inn blended the indoors with the outdoors.

My son-in-law needed to leave for Europe on July 26. I'd promised to take care of my granddaughter Chrissie while Steve was in Europe. And I still had Guam and Hawaii to travel—I was running out of time. My hostess at the inn called a businessman down the street, then we went together to his home. Mr. Sugimoto had a lengthy phone conversation with Mrs. Ueda in Yokohama (my next contact stop). He then called the bullet train to see if they would allow me to take my bike on board.

Yes, they would! We jumped into his van. When we arrived at the train station, they didn't want to take the bike on the fast passenger train. Mr. Sugimoto pleaded my case, and again they relented. We hurried to catch the train. Thanks to the stationmaster, ticket agents, Mr. Sugimoto, and I'll never know who else, they got me to the platform on time. A stately gentleman, Mr. Statematsu, spoke to me in English and sat with me in the special compartment the bike was assigned to.

"Years ago I went to New York and Americans were very helpful," he said. "I want to help you in return."

When the train stopped, the chief controller, dressed in a white suit, stepped out, picked up the bike, then turned and boarded the streamliner. We hurried on behind him, and the train was on its way. In Yokohama, the controller again stepped in, picked up the bike, and carried it to the platform.

Pastor Ueda, his son, and daughter came to pick me up in Yokohama. On Sabbath I spoke briefly in two of the services at church. That afternoon the editor of the *Signs of the Times* magazine interviewed me and took some pictures. He then took me to the Tokyo hospital compound with another editor. I had a call from Shuko Ogawa, the journalist I had met in Thailand. She took me to dinner the next day and gave me a copy of the *Update,* a magazine that seemed to be mostly about people in different countries, and how they lived.

Pastor Nishiura took me to catch the limousine to the airport. We arrived and purchased a ticket, then discovered they wouldn't take the bicycle in the limousine. The pastor got a refund on the ticket, but what should we do now? Drive all the way to the Tokyo station and see if they could get it on there? Again I prayed for God's help.

A short time later we heard the welcome words "You can take

the bike." The pastor went back and bought the ticket again, and the driver put my wheels in the back of the baggage compartment. "If we have a lot of luggage to pick up in Tokyo we might have to do something else with it," he warned. But he never even stopped in Tokyo. We went right on to the airport. Apparently no one else needed his services to get to the airport.

THE ISLANDS OF THE SEA

At the airport I confirmed my ticket to Guam. I started for the gate, which was some distance away, then realized the ticket agent had made the ticket for the bike out for Karachi, Pakistan. I ran back toward the security desk. There on the wall was a phone. "Please, be sure that my bike is ticketed to Guam," I said in Japanese and English.

. The agent assured me they had corrected the error. My Japanese isn't very fluent, but I had made my point, perhaps with only seconds to spare before I boarded.

We landed in Guam in midafternoon. The hot, humid air felt suffocating, but the beauty of the place outweighed the unpleasant atmosphere. I called Pastor Jimeno, who came right away. He was the same caring person I remembered from long ago when I was a missionary there with my family. Pastor Jimeno took me to a modern apartment in Agana, the location of our church headquarters. The apartment had cooking facilities and air-conditioning.

Next he handed me a schedule that didn't seem to allow time for eating and sleeping. I could fit most of it in, but I had to remember that I was here to ride the length of the island and then be on my way to Hawaii. The next morning I left with Mary Ellen, the young lady responsible for working with the media on my behalf, to bike to the south end of the island. Agana was in the middle of the island. I planned to ride south first, and north later.

After an hour, as we came into a little village, a large nail punctured the tire on Mary Ellen's bicycle. We tried to telephone someone for assistance, but without success. After 30 minutes I decided it was best that I continue on without her. The commissioner of the village took Mary Ellen back to Agana to the bike shop.

The road was so steep that I walked and pushed my cycle a lot of the way. The temperature was only about 85°F., but the humidity took my breath away. One hill I climbed must have been four miles long. Mary Ellen caught up with me in another village. I wanted to know if this was really the end of the island and learned that a little farther on actually was. After another hour or so we had gone past it. Pastor Willie arrived to take us back.

Two newspapers interviewed me in the afternoon, then I attended a meeting to plan the big parade for Thursday, July 21, celebrating Liberation Day. The next day I literally hit the road running: a TV interview at 8:00, an interview with the governor at 10:00, a noon visit to the new mission clinic, and then off at 1:45 to the northern part of the island to bike back to Agana.

Pastor Jimeno took me to the front entrance of the large armed forces installation that occupies the northern tip of the island. An Air Force truck took me to the back of their property, as far as the road went. I started my bicycle ride at that point with a police escort to the front gate. A TV reporter took pictures of me leaving the base. I thought I would be alone on the ride back to Agana, but a young man named Steve arrived to accompany me. We made the 18-mile trip in an hour and 15 minutes.

That evening at prayer meeting I spoke about the miracles of God's grace in preserving my life as I journeyed through many parts of the globe. On Thursday we enjoyed the Liberation Day celebration. Parade floats were fashioned from palm branches, flowers, and long grasses cleverly woven together. Everyone had prepared great quantities of food. Any celebration gets a lot of cooperation from the Guamanian people. Jimenos fixed a picnic lunch and took me to the park. Later we visited American World Radio with its six high towers and modern, powerful equipment that beams a message of hope to Europe, South America, and many parts of Asia.

Before I knew it, I was on my way to another island—Hawaii. I landed in Honolulu on the island of Oahu early in the morning. The governor had sent Florence Tsany from the visitors' information program at the airport to help me through customs. Cecilia Seabury (who had been my support driver through Europe), her two children who lived on the island, and Janine Youngberg, a student nurse I had taught at Andrews, came to greet me. I received several welcoming leis, including one from the governor. Shirley Goodrich took me to her house, where I would stay while in Hawaii. A journalist from the Honolulu *Star-Bulletin* arrived to interview me, as did Channel 4, and KIVT had my story live on the noon news.

Janine and I tried bicycling around the city but felt uncomfortable in the traffic. We gave up the idea of cycling and went swimming instead. Shirley took me for a ride after church the next day, and in the evening I spoke at vespers in Kailua.

Kathy and Cecilia flew with me to the island of Hawaii the next morning. The plane landed at 7:00, and I was out on the road by 8:00. My route included lots of climbing and rolling hills. Other than that, I had good roads and beautiful scenery to enjoy as I rode. I covered nearly 63 miles. That night Kathy drove us to her cabin, built in a bed of lava on top of the mountain. She had to transport water to the cabin, but the beauty of the surroundings compensated for any inconvenience. Cecilia and I slept on mats that night.

The next day I kept climbing for about eight miles. As I faced the strongest head winds of the entire trip so far, I wondered if I should turn around and go north. But I felt impressed to continue south, and later considered that one of the most important answers to prayer on the entire trip. Had I turned and gone the other way, I don't know how I would have found Cecilia or the airport later in the day.

Before long, I reached the other side of the mountain and enjoyed a wonderful downhill grade. When I came to Panaluu Park, I went to look for Cecilia and Kathy at our planned meeting place by the Black Sands Beach. And there they were! We enjoyed a picnic lunch together, and then the girls left me to finish the last 10 miles to the airport. When I landed in Honolulu, I biked the short distance to the other airport, where I would leave at 9:15 for home. It was aloha time once more.

I arrived in Chicago the next afternoon and took a short hop across Lake Michigan to South Bend, Indiana. My arrival hadn't been announced, and I appreciated the chance to get my feet on the ground first. I wondered if Gene (who had been afraid he would never see me again) would be there to meet me. I needn't have worried. The sight of his familiar face helped to erase all those lonesome hours away from home.

A journalist from the South Bend *Tribune* arrived to take pictures. A large picture of Gene welcoming me appeared the next day in the South Bend paper. The leis around my neck seemed a fitting symbol of love, happiness, and unity around the whole earth.

There was so much catching up to do. I found out that son-in-law Steve couldn't go to Europe after all, so I could have taken a little longer on the last lap of the journey if I had called home sooner. When I called my daughter, Ladonna, in Washington, she was eager to tell me all the things I had missed while I was away. "Please, hurry and come see me, Mom!" she pleaded. My family in Canada were also happy to know that I was safe at home again.

A homecoming parade was scheduled for Thursday in Berrien Springs. I needed to get a haircut, go through the stack of mail on my desk, and settle back into a daily routine. After spending some time with my family, I must ride 1,000 miles in British Columbia to make up for the miles lost in China and elsewhere in Asia.

1,000 MILES TO MY 70TH BIRTHDAY

I was on the road again in the Mini-Cruiser. Blanche, who had driven across part of America with me, joined me. We visited Ladonna in Seattle for a few days, then continued on to Qualicum Beach on Vancouver Island, where my brother and sister lived. George's garden provided a feast of fresh vegetables, and Marion's flowers provided a feast for our eyes.

The next day we headed north to Port Hardy, the northernmost town on the island. George asked me why I picked British

Columbia as the place to make up miles since it was, in his words, "just one big hill."

"Well, brother," I told him, "a magnet drew me over to where you chose to hang out, and I just felt this was as good as any place to begin."

A lot had happened since the day Marion and I had said good-bye at Oceanside. I'd been a little fearful then. Now I felt confident I could do almost anything if I tried. The trip from Port Hardy south to Victoria would cover about 300 miles. I made 65 miles the first day, which included lots of climbing. *Oh, why didn't I choose Nebraska?* I joked with myself.

I stopped each day at noon to pray for a safe place to park for the night. By the time we got to the rest stop at Roberts Lake we still hadn't located a suitable place. Then three young people came along and remarked, "Why, there's a place right around the corner at the store." God continued to provide all that we needed on our journey.

We wanted to get back to Qualicum Beach before the weekend so we would miss the heavy Labor Day traffic. On the last day my meter read 72 miles when I stopped cycling in late afternoon. We still had 19.2 miles to go to the end of the ride and would have to return on Sunday to my stopping point and finish the last 20 miles.

I spoke at the church in Nanaimo the next day, and we spent the afternoon in a park, refreshing our minds and our spirits.

It took me two hours on Monday to ride from my Friday stopping point back into Qualicum Beach. I stopped long enough to say goodbye to George and Marion. "I'll see you in Kelowna on the 27th," I told them.

George begged me not to be on the road on Sunday and Monday. "There's so much drinking," he said, "and so many people from the mainland come to the island for Labor Day weekend."

"I'll come back if it looks like trouble out there," I promised.

The roads became better, with fewer hills, but I couldn't deny that the traffic was very heavy. I was quite a ways down the road when I came upon an accident scene that I haven't been able to forget. A car had struck a cyclist, severely injuring him and making a pretzel of his bike. White bread in a wrapper, a sleeping bag, clothes, and a blood-stained towel littered the side of the road. Had I not already traveled so many miles I probably would have turned back.

When Blanche and I stopped at a fruit stand along the road, the lady proprietor insisted that I accept a gift of $10. Although I wasn't raising money on the road, if someone wanted to help a little I didn't stop them. Later that evening we pulled into a camp for the night. I was almost out of Canadian money, and there was no place to cash a travelers check. So the lady's $10 saved the day! My meter indicated we had covered 60 miles. The next day we rode into Victoria, where we enjoyed a short visit with Doug and Lucy, Marion's son and daughter-in-law, and their family. We spent the night with Helen and Frank White. She and I had been roommates 40 years before.

I saw snowcapped Mount Baker the next morning, dominating the skyline across the border. The scene reminded me of the psalmist's declaration "I will look to the hills from whence cometh my strength" (Ps. 121:1). We stopped at Hope to visit the facility where seminars, camp meetings, and health programs take place. At Alpine Camp, east of Boston Bar, the rain poured down. Until then, the only place the rain had dictated what I must do was in Japan.

We rode through Fraser Canyon beside the Fraser River on Highway 97 north. I wanted to go as far as Hudson Hope by the Peace River, quite a way north of Prince George. We decided to drive up, and then I would ride my bicycle back to Cache Creek. On our way south again we enjoyed the fall colors. The leaves were turning from pale green to dark green to yellow and orange, and the forest appeared to be on fire with color. I had bicycled 55 miles by 7:00 p.m., and we stopped overnight at an antique shop. The owners allowed us to use their backyard and invited us to stay for breakfast.

I faced a strong head wind over Pine Pass the next day, but still made 59 miles. That evening I called Ladonna. She planned to come up by bus, meet us at Cache Creek, and help out the last week on the road. I counted the days until her arrival.

Back on the road after supper, I made excellent time. This part of the world was almost uninhabited. A man at the ski station told

Blanche there wasn't a phone or a place to stay for 30 miles. I felt impressed to go on, and Blanche followed close behind. I knew it was risky to be out so late, but I hated to backtrack and lose time.

We were in bear country. I told Blanche that if one ever took out after me she must get a good picture of the two of us! As I came around a bend in the road I spotted a highway maintenance camp. A young man there said that campers and RVs often stopped overnight in the summer. He showed us where to hook up our camper and offered us the use of the showers.

We stopped at the Provincial Park the next night. They had just closed the park for the day and shut off the water, so staying overnight would be free. After dinner, however, a forest ranger came over and told us the government employees were going on strike. We must leave the park. Fortunately, a homeowner nearby allowed us to hook up next to his house for the night. The nights had gotten very cold, and we left the camper's electric heater on all night.

We arrived in Prince George on Sunday and spent the night with Pastor Wells and his family. (Pastor Wells was the Seventh-day Adventist pastor in Prince George. He and his family were a great help to us while we were there.) The next day I spoke at the school and had three interviews—newspaper, television and radio. I was covering between 50 and 68 miles a day and didn't mind the crisp, cool air; actually, I found it very invigorating.

The next night we hooked up at the home of a lovely Lutheran lady named Goldie Bakers. She invited us in for a visit, and some of her neighbors stopped in while we were there. They entertained us with bear stories, including one about coming home and finding a bear trying to get in the window. They told us that banging two rocks together, or shouting, will sometimes drive the bear away. That night I had dreams of bears trying to get in the windows of our camper.

Two more days until Ladonna would arrive! I didn't want to be late to meet her bus. The next night we stopped at the home of a kindly man who lived in a little house with 17 cats. I'm not sure what he did to make ends meet, but there surely were a lot of cats who were thankful he was around.

We reached Williams Lake about 6:30 the following evening. Harry Bechtold came by. He and his wife, Audrey, had been my classmates 50 years before. We recognized each other instantly. He asked me to speak in prayer meeting that night. Although pressed for time, I did speak to the group, then hurried away to pick up Ladonna at the bus station. We got there just as the bus arrived. The three of us stayed up talking until 1:00 in the morning. I was so happy that Ladonna would be with me when I completed 8,000 miles on my 70th birthday!

It was snowing when we headed south for the 100-mile house. In earlier days, these mile houses had been stopping places along Highway 97 for stage coaches. We came across a trailer that had flipped over in the road and scattered its contents in all directions. Ladonna stopped and helped to direct traffic.

That afternoon I got wet and became chilled as I rode. Slush covered the ground and a wet snow continued to fall. Many small trees bent almost to the ground from a five-inch snow that had fallen a week before. We made it to the 88-mile house that evening and hooked up behind a log cabin restaurant. The temperature outside was 34°F.

The next day was our rest day. We walked, read, and visited with the people in the cabin. That evening Ladonna decided we needed some popcorn. Apparently, we put too many kernels in the pan. The popcorn quickly filled the pan up to the lid. When I lifted the lid just a fraction of an inch, the popping corn knocked the lid completely off the pan. Popcorn hit the ceiling and walls, and some even landed in Ladonna's hair. We ate it anyway.

The next morning Cecilia and Ladonna both expressed reluctance about traveling because of the weather. I didn't want to put them in danger, but somehow I knew everything would be all right. "I have only today, then Vernon to Kelowna tomorrow and I'll be done," I urged. "I must fill the remaining gap to Cache Creek." I started out in the wrong direction and didn't discover my mistake until I had covered nine miles in the slush. I wanted to cry. Fortunately, a man and his son stopped when I showed signs of needing help. They picked me up and drove back over the nine

Ride With the Wind

miles. When we reached the 88-mile house we measured nine miles in the correct direction and I resumed my journey.

Ladonna and Cecilia reached the motel in Cache Creek first. A number of people had gathered to give me a big hurrah when I arrived. A large picture of the three of us accompanied the article in the newspaper the next day. I finished my trip at Cache Creek, and I did ride from Vernon to Kelowna, making up some of the miles I had lost in Asia. The next day we rode by car through Kamloops, stopping in Armstrong to visit an old friend before we were on our way again, following the lakes and hills to Vernon. My sister's son, who lived in Vernon, took me to dinner. But by 3:00 I was back on the cycle, following Okanagan Lake toward Kelowna. That night my older brother, Arthur Patterson; his wife, Kay; my younger brother, George; my sister, Marion; Ladonna; Blanche; and I all went to the Peaches Restaurant for supper.

The next day would be my 70th birthday. Marion and I stopped at the hospital (where I had been born) to check out the plans for the grand finale of my trip. At 1:00 I started across Okanagan Lake on the longest floating bridge in the world. (I had wanted to swim across, but it was too late in the season.) Two television stations, three newspapers, and two radio stations covered the finish of my journey. Speeches, flowers, and the presentation of gifts completed the celebration. This was the first time Ladonna could be with me on such an occasion. I hoped she knew how very much it meant to have my only daughter there to celebrate with me. The family celebrated together that evening. Pink roses, a birthday cake, and everything that loved ones do for each other finished out the day.

Was this the end, or was there more to come? Yes, much more!

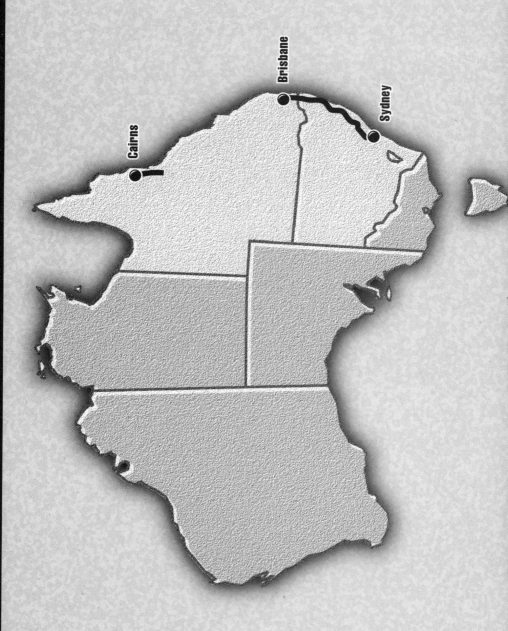

Cairns

Brisbane

Sydney

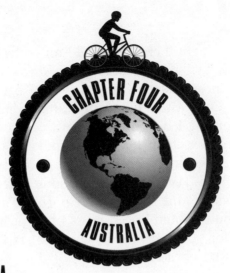

CHAPTER FOUR

AUSTRALIA

BEAUTIFUL AUSTRALIA

I landed in Cairns, on the northeastern shore of Australia, on August 11, 1992. Pastor Ross Baines welcomed me at the airport and saw me safely off on my way south. The Australian Conference of Seventh-day Adventists had arranged for people to meet me along the route. These contact people, most of whom I had never met, helped me get my wheels on the ground, as it were. As always, starting a new trip produced a few anxious moments. Alone, with no knowledge of the roads, traffic, or people, I again put my trust in my unseen Guide.

I rode across roads that were very narrow and rough in places and had a hard time climbing the hills. It felt like something on the bike was not balanced properly. However, the countryside was beautiful and the mountains lush with greenery. Sugar cane towered 15 feet high on either side of the road. People interested in what I was doing offered assistance along the way, each adding to the joy of my trip. One woman gave me a pair of sunglasses, and a cordial bank owner cashed a traveler's check for me.

I encountered few cyclists on the road, but that first afternoon I shared a discussion with three of them (two Americans and a Canadian, all men) about which routes to take and where to stay. The two Americans planned to sleep in the Australian bush. The small town of Mirriwinni would be my last chance to find accommodations for the night. I chalked off 43 miles the first day and felt surprisingly spry. Lynne and Eddie Pryor, owners of a craft store, offered me their hospitality. I enjoyed a "spit" bath in the laundry tub and slept in a bed with a billowing feather comforter on top.

The next morning I bought some soya cheese and mixed nuts from a little store next door. Everyone I spoke to thought I should take the train to Rockhampton and start my trip from there. Otherwise, they said, I would encounter long miles of uninhabited territory. But water and help would both be available on the Rockhampton route should I need it. As I left for Innisfail 14 miles away, I prayed for guidance about where to start. I had to be in Sydney in a month to head for home.

In Innisfail I discovered that the trains ran only twice a week. So I left on the evening bus. A full moon lit up the landscape. From my window seat I could see the rubber plantations and lush growth along the road. The bus driver advised me to go on to Brisbane, then ride to Sydney from there. He said the roads from Rockhampton to Brisbane were narrow and dangerous, with few accommodations available. When I arrived in Rockhampton the next morning, someone quickly helped me get a ticket so that the bus for Brisbane wouldn't leave without me.

Windmills occasionally dotted the bare landscape. As the bus rolled along on the narrow roads, the driver and a passenger, who was also a bus driver, did their best to scare me off the road. "As many as 300 kangaroos are killed out here every night. Often they are hit and knocked off the road and the driver never even stops. You could be one of those animals and we'd never know the difference. And who knows when or where you would be found?" the driver said.

When we arrived in Brisbane, a young man helped me call Aussie Way Backpackers Hostel. They sent a young girl to pick me up, and I slept safely that night in my room at the hostel. At breakfast the next morning, I enjoyed a conversation with Michael Gay. He said he was trying to live a good life and search for peace at the same time. We talked about adventure and everyday things. When we parted I felt that perhaps I'd had a part in helping him through that archway where serenity, acceptance, and a little faith worked their way into his heart. He saw me in town later and thanked me for helping him find hope and new meaning in his life.

The main road was across the city on the outskirts of Brisbane. So I rode the local train to Beenleigh, ate the lunch I'd brought along, and was back on my bicycle on the road south. Something *was* wrong with the bicycle. It was still quite difficult to turn my pedals on the hills. I went back to Beenleigh. The manager of the Beenleigh Cycle Shop realized immediately that the front wheel brake needed adjusting, and I was soon on my way again.

The traffic was fairly heavy and the road offered very little shoulder. Then the bicycle wheel turned off the pavement and I fell in deep shale. A young mother passing by stopped to help me. Although my ankle hurt I felt I could continue. In Coomera I contacted Dr. Karl Marzini, who came over to the hardware store where I had stopped and whisked my bike and me to Dreamtime Caravan Park. He paid for one night's lodging and later brought over a tasty dish his wife had prepared. Dr. Marzini operated a natural therapies clinic in Coomera, using natural methods to treat chronic diseases, such as diabetes. He and I were definitely on the same frequency. My ankle bothered me some during the night, so I took a Motrin and finally drifted off to sleep.

At church the next day I gave a short talk on my life of adventure and hoped my comments started some people thinking about taking responsibility for making things right in their lives. The Marzinis invited me for dinner after church, and I enjoyed the opportunity to hear more success stories from the work of the clinic.

As I was ready to leave Sunday morning, I noticed the pressure was down in one of the bicycle tires. The tire wouldn't inflate when I added air. A young man in the caravan park stopped to look at it for me, discovered a split inside the valve, and put in a new tube. I thought of all the miles I'd traveled where assistance was not available, only to have a flat tire on the doorstep of someone who could help me.

On the road I met Laurence and Stella Lonergan. They advised me to reroute and take the alternate road in order to miss the high pass over the hills. They even took me to the place I needed to start. In Brunswick Head I discovered there were no hostels in the area. A woman in the pharmacy where I stopped to ask about accommodations knew an Adventist couple and called them on my behalf. They not only invited me to spend the night with them, but even came to the pharmacy to pick me up. In Australia Seventh-day Adventists are well known for their hospitals and for the health food industry they operate, which is the largest in the country.

My message on health travels fastest through the media. On the way to Ballina, Fay Clissold at the tourist office called ABC radio at Byron Bay, who interviewed me over the phone. During the afternoon a TV crew showed up, asked the usual questions, and made a videotape of me riding along the road, a clip that aired over NBN that night.

In Ballina I stayed in a backpacker's cabin. The warm comforter really helped as the night was very cold. While my right ankle still swelled during the day, the swelling went down when I rested at night.

The terrain changed day by day. I entered flatter country, and then more rolling hills. The dark green countryside looked so healthy. I enjoyed lunch in Woodburn, which had the most colorful and elegant display of fresh food I had ever seen. Bright oranges, green peppers, yellow this, and red that—a feast for the eye as well as the body. I rested for a while, then headed out again.

Someone told me I could make it to a caravan park up the road before dark. I rode on and on, seeing nothing but heavy forest on both sides of the narrow, winding road. (I was so thankful the bicycle tube had not waited until now to split.) Just as I began to wonder if I would have to sleep in the bush, a big sign proclaimed: Woombah Woods Park Village. The only heat in the place were the hot plates on the stove, so I was cold most of the night. But at least I was inside.

Finding drinking water sometimes presented a problem. I needed to drink often to prevent dehydration. Sometimes I drank right out of rain barrels and tanks that collected water runoff from roofs. In some countries it would have been a foolish thing to do, but I never got sick from this in Australia. I enjoyed lunch at a small farm that grew more than two dozen fruit trees on its small acreage.

As I hurried to get to Grafton before sunset, I passed egrets eating in the fields. Magpies rested on the fenceposts, and blue herons flew ahead of me as if they were guiding me south to my destination. That night I stayed at 200-year-old Rathgan House. The windows didn't have locks; anyone could have climbed through from the porch outside. *God has taken care of me this long,* I thought, *why would He change now?*

By Friday, August 21, I was on my way to Woolgoolga, after being on a live broadcast from one of the radio stations in Grafton in the morning. When people began tooting their horns as they passed, it encouraged me to know they wished me well. Two more weeks and I would be on my way home!

This was banana country. Great banana groves covered the hills. When I stopped at the Going Bananas Motel to use the phone, someone called Norma Pink, who lived nearby. She came and whisked me off to her country home for a huge dinner. I spent two nights with Norma, her husband, John, and their son. We went to Coffs Harbor church on the Pacific Highway, where I met Prim Sisk. Prim was a nurse at Loma Linda, California, where I had trained so many years before. A Mrs. Atchison interviewed me for the newspaper, and Dot Connor, who lived 32 miles away, invited me to spend the next night with her. However, I planned to be much farther down the road by bedtime on Sunday.

Back on the road, Dr. John Dulhunty and his family stopped me for a visit. (I had stayed with his brother Paul and family in Katmandu, Nepal.) I spent the night with a family in Nambucca Heads and was on the road again by 8:20 the following morning. I had traveled about an hour when Paul Gallagher from *Guardian News* stopped me and asked for an interview, which I was happy to do. (I had already given a phone interview before leaving Nambucca Heads.)

I passed through Macksville, then ate dinner beside a river. I planned to stay with Pastor Tulevu's family in Kempsey, but realized I couldn't reach Kempsey before dark. The manager's wife at a travel stop took me to their home, where I was warmly welcomed by this marvelous family.

The next morning my host family helped me get back to where I had stopped the night before. As soon as I rode into the wind I knew it was in control, not I. After fighting my way forward for three hours and covering only eight miles, I decided to stop and wait for the wind to calm. I finally reached Kempsey by midafternoon and went to the Willow Brook Caravan Park to get a room for the night.

My ankle continued to bother me (I suspected I had broken a small bone on top of my foot); however, I wouldn't be able to manage a cast, even if I needed one. So I'd just have to be very careful to keep the foot aligned properly on the pedal.

The deadline for finishing the trip drew closer every day. The next two days I made about 30 miles before lunch. Pastor and Mrs. Sanders offered me their hospitality in Kew. I was thankful once more for the opportunity to meet such wonderful Christian people who believed in the golden rule.

The weather was great and my energy level high as I made my way through a number of small towns along the way. Sometimes people who had seen me on TV stopped me to chat for a few moments or to take a picture. One evening I was having difficulty in finding a place to sleep for the night. I stopped at a store just before closing time. The manager told me that road construction crews had taken every available accommodation. Several nearby houses had lights in their windows. I wondered if anyone out there would take someone in who was wearing a helmet and riding a bike. A man who had come into the store for supplies overheard the manager tell me there might be something farther ahead over the hill. By now it was truly dark outside.

"I'm Allen," the man introduced himself. "I'll go up the hill and check to see if anything at all is available."

He returned in a few minutes with a smile on his face.

"You're smiling," I said. "You must have good news."

"No," he replied, "there's nothing at the hotel, and you can't stay in the bunkhouse with the men. But I'm going to let you stay in my caravan for tonight. I'll go up to the bunkhouse and spend the night there with the other men."

He took me over to his place and told me to help myself to anything in the refrigerator, and even use his sleeping bag. Some women would be petrified to accept such an offer. He had the keys to the place and said he'd come by in the morning to pick up his work clothes. But I had prayed about the whole matter. Maybe *he* was the one taking a risk by inviting a total stranger to use his living quarters for the night! I found out later he was the superintendent of the crew working on the road. I shall always be grateful for that warm shelter that night.

RUDE AWAKENING

Raindrops began to fall from angry, dark clouds. I took shelter on a farmer's front porch. When the elements calmed down, I wondered what to do next. It was dangerous to ride in such weather. I found a fruit stand around the next bend in the road. Colin, the owner, offered to store my bike in his shed.

"I'll run you down to Bulahdelah, on the other side of the mountain," he said. "On second thought, here comes the mail carrier. She's going right your way."

I would just have to have faith that somehow I could get back to this place on Sunday morning to get my bike. The closest accommodations were Alum Mountain Caravan Park. I enjoyed the opportunity to get organized, have something to eat, and go to bed early. I kept my housecoat on for added warmth.

The rattling of the door at 2:00 a.m. woke me out of a sound sleep. The whole travel trailer swayed back and forth. Then the door gave way and a very tall young man came in and stood like a statue next to the table. I can move pretty fast in the short sprints, so I charged by him and out the door. A middle-aged man leaned against his car at another caravan across the way. Now I was in the middle with two men to contend with.

"Can't you see that someone has broken into my trailer?" I asked the man by the car. "Come and help me!" By then I could tell that both were quite drunk. When the younger man came out of my trailer, I darted back in and locked the door (which didn't mean much). I grabbed my emergency whistle and blew three strong blasts several times. It must have made a small impression in the men's reasoning powers, because the man by my door finally went over to the other trailer. Then the older man came up to the door and wanted to come inside.

"Go on home to bed *now!*" I commanded. Everything became very quiet. *Should I go up to headquarters?* I wondered. If I did, the men might get in my trailer and lock me outside. I prayed for protection and went to sleep.

The next morning Don and Olive Shepherd picked me up and took me to church. When I returned to the park in the afternoon, I met the older of the two men from the night before. He informed me that "A drunk broke into my mother's place one night, and when she saw he was drunk she just laughed."

"Frankly, I can't see anything funny about someone breaking into my quarters at 2:00 in the morning," I told him. "Be sure it doesn't happen again tonight."

Alcohol is one of man's worst enemies. It has been suggested that a drink or two of wine each day is helpful in preventing heart attacks. I wonder how many people, especially young people, use this as an excuse to drink. The truth is that unfermented grape juice or artificially dried raisins offer some of the same benefits with none of the bad effects.

The Shepherds returned me to the fruit stand where I had left my bike on Friday. Don wanted me to put my bike in his pickup and ride over the top in the truck. "It's one of the most dangerous highways anywhere—steep hills, sharp corners—you can't see what's on the other side," he worried. "Semis take all the road."

"I can't ride," I told him. "I must go over that mountain under my own power." I knew that yielding once could open the door to do it anytime the going got a little rough. It wouldn't be truthful to say that I wasn't a bit worried myself. Still, I felt everything would turn out all right. I picked up my gear and was on my way.

Because it was Sunday there was less traffic. The roads were good and everyone gave me room. I spent about five-and-a-half hours walking and climbing to the summit. It took only half an hour to go down the other side. George and Linda Drinkall were watching for me on the road. George, who was health and communications director for the North New South Wales Conference, had been in on some of the plans made in my behalf. We had a pleasant visit before they went on their way.

The Atcheson family, who had passed me earlier, drove up again with refreshments and encouragement. Mrs. Atcheson wrote in my log: "May God continue to protect this fantastic lady."

Rain threatened again. I looked for a place to stop and wait out the approaching storm. A winding dirt road led me through some trees into a little settlement in the woods. I saw a horse and cow, but no people. As I ate under the shelter of a shed, little rivers of rain ran off the roof. With some anxiety, I watched for someone to open a door or appear from somewhere. When the rain stopped, I got my things together and hurried back out to the winding road. That night, safe and dry at Karuah Caravan Park, I laughed at the howling wind that shook the walls. This would be home for the night.

I had to make my decision quickly. Should I go by Newcastle and down through the winding roads by the sea, or farther inland to Kurri Kurri and south to Avondale? I decided to go inland. Strong winds buffeted me as I rode. That afternoon the Raymond *Terrace* interviewed me and took pictures for their paper. Then I bought some food, a new tube for my bike, and cashed some traveler's checks. Back on the road I fought the wind every inch of the way. After 23 miles I stopped at Ponderosa Caravan Park in Tomago.

George Drinkall took me to Newcastle for a TV interview before I left the next day. NBN did a long interview and filmed me riding the bicycle. These journalists and other media representatives were often interested in what I was doing. Sometimes we had long talks on what a gift good health is.

I arrived at the little town of Kurri Kurri that evening. The town didn't have a hostel, but a man told me of a motel at the top of the hill. "It will cost you $40 to stay there," he said.

I definitely was not interested in climbing any more hills *or* in paying $40.

"Right across the street is a pub," the man added. "They have rooms upstairs for wayfarers. It's safe and clean. Australia has these pubs all over. We have a saying that if a stranger comes through town, give him a drink and a bed for the night."

I didn't feel a need for the drink but could surely use the bed. I went to the pub and sat down at the bar, as if I had control of the situation.

"What would you like to drink?" asked the bartender.

"Could you give me a cup of hot water?"

By now eyes from all four directions had turned toward me, and everyone strained to hear what would happen next. A tall, blond middle-aged man walked up to the bar. "Here's a $50 bill. Give this lady anything she wants."

I told him thank you, but I didn't drink. Then I quietly began to plan my escape. "I hear you have rooms for rent here."

"Yes, they're $10." (I learned later that the rooms were really $20, but someone had already passed the other $10 under the counter.)

After I settled in I went down to see if the evening news was covering my story. I seldom had the opportunity to watch the news, so it was a real treat to see the interview. The whole place was very old and faded. I had a soak in the deep, old-fashioned tub down the hall and went to bed early. Someone had brought a heavy comforter which kept me warm throughout the night.

I passed near Avondale College the next day and debated whether I should take time to visit it. I decided to take the road to Avondale. I had turned off the road to Cooranbong when a man driving a semi stopped along the road.

"Hello!" he called. "I heard over the radio that we truck drivers are your guardian angels."

"Yes, you're right," I smiled back. "I know that if I'm ever in danger or hurt that any of you will help me out."

"How about me putting your bike in and giving you a ride to the top of the hill?" he offered.

"You know that I would if I could, but my conscience would

bother me. As much as I'd like to, I must go on under my own steam." I thanked him for stopping, and watched him speed up the road ahead of me.

The freeway had less traffic and long stretches of nothing but cattle ranches and wide, open fields. I finally arrived at the Avondale campus and received a royal welcome. I stayed overnight and found everyone to be helpful and accommodating.

Avondale College started around the turn of the century. Ellen White, a dedicated leader in the early days of the Adventist Church, received a vision that this particular property was the place to locate the school. People considered the soil useless for growing food, but Mrs. White insisted that this was the place. The land turned out to be very productive, surpassing anyone's dreams, for raising crops and supplying pasture for animals. Students worked for their tuition, learning more than what was taught in books. The school is a place that cherishes honesty, integrity, and hard work.

Before I resumed my journey the next day, I visited the Australian home of Ellen White, who had written, among many other things, about health. In her later years she went to Australia. Through her influence a productive program of education, health, and spiritual guidance was developed that has become one of the largest health food industries in the world.

I wanted to see how far I could ride toward my Sydney finish line before dark. People stopped me on four different occasions to chat and share their stories. What a day! Then it started to rain. Again. I took an off-ramp into Industrial City. There I learned that it was too far to get to Sydney before dark. I was thankful the rain had caused me to stop for the night.

There were no overnight accommodations in the city, so I phoned Mrs. Madden, my contact in the area, who lived about 25 miles away. She contacted the Cliffords, who lived somewhat closer. Mrs. Clifford called and gave me directions on how to find their place. It turned out to be quite some distance, but the roads were smooth and easy to travel. The Cliffords, retired missionaries, did everything possible to give me a proper send-off to Sydney the next morning. Mr. Clifford helped me find the right road on the map, and his wife packed a sandwich for me to eat along the way. (He checked later to see if I had arrived.)

About 12:30 I saw a sign: End of Freeway. I had almost completed my long trek. It really hadn't been that hard. I'd enjoyed breath-taking scenery, friendly people, and many happy hours on the road.

When I reached Pacific Highway, I followed the signs to Sydney Adventist Hospital. This beautiful landmark, loved by the Australian people because the staff genuinely cares about them, made me proud to be a nurse. I faxed a message from the hospital to let my family know that I had arrived. Dr. Butler, from the division office, took me to the home of Ethel Brethowser, where I spent four glorious days before flying back to the United States.

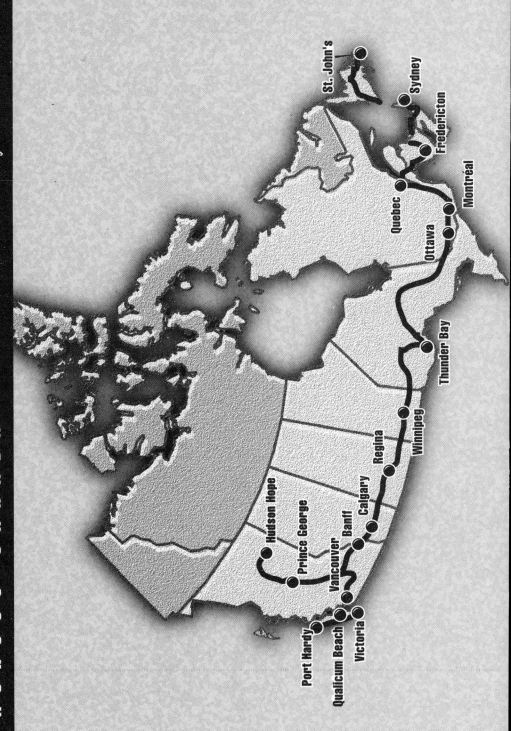

ACROSS CANADA

July 7 – October 12, 1993

St. John's
Sydney
Fredericton
Montréal
Quebec
Ottawa
Thunder Bay
Winnipeg
Regina
Calgary
Banff
Vancouver
Hudson Hope
Prince George
Port Hardy
Qualicum Beach
Victoria

CHAPTER FIVE

CANADA

CBC MOVIE SEND-OFF

At the ripe young age of 74, I was about to begin the longest trek of my life. I planned to ride my bicycle 4,000 miles across the Trans-Canada Highway, the longest paved road in the world. My son, Gene, would accompany me and wear all the hats—driver, cook, media director, photographer, manager, and whatever else it would take to get me from one side of the continent to the other.

Just before we left Gene had me practicing on roller blades before the camera started to roll for a WNDU interview. All went well until I hit a pothole that immediately stopped me dead in my tracks. I must have broken a rib or two, so my chest was sore when we began our journey.

We said goodbye to friends and family and headed for Vancouver, British Columbia. That first night we parked at the home of my niece and her husband, Patty and Jim Howden. Jim helped us catch the ferry for Vancouver Island the next day. Just as we got on the ferry I remembered I had left our money, traveler's checks, and my shoes in the RV. Gene ran back to get them and hopped back on the ferry just as the gangplank was going up.

We spent a wonderful Fourth of July weekend on Vancouver Island with my brother, sister, and other family members. On Wednesday, July 7, we were on our way at last. First, though, we had a big date with CBC down at the water's edge in Crescent

Beach. The interview lasted several hours while the crew video-taped me riding the bike. I gave them still pictures that had been taken of my bike trips in other countries. Then we headed to Vinier Park that overlooks the planetarium in downtown Vancouver. CBC came back for a few more shots, and two radio stations, The Vancouver Province and J. R. Country, conducted interviews. After supper I put my hand in the water of Crescent Beach and we were officially underway. We reached Langley by 9:00 p.m. and spent the night in a Mennonite church lot.

We arrived in Cache Creek late the next day. (I had covered most of this section before.) After interviews for the evening news, I began to realize that I would need to budget my time with the media if I was going to keep on schedule. Because winter arrives early in some of the northern provinces, I had to complete my trip in October and must pace myself accordingly. So despite the lateness of the hour, I started east toward Kamloops. The mountains towered above me on my right. How much I had missed them! I'd been born about 100 miles south of where I now rode. I knew this country would always be a part of me, and I wanted to find a way to spend more time in these wonderful hills.

We started across a barren desert of sagebrush, sand, desert plants, and hills that were as bald as the wilderness, an unchanging landscape that stretched on for miles. When I began riding early the next morning we were still in the desert, but now the wide Thompson River ran through the middle of the panoramic view. I could see there would be lots of climbing. I was traveling down a steep hill at 38 miles an hour and couldn't see the bridge that lay around a sharp corner at the bottom of the hill until I was on it. The bridge, constructed of a lattice-like metal, was wet and slippery. All I could do was cling to my wide antler handlebars with all my strength, aware that the smallest slip could send me hurtling who knows where. *God, help me make it across this long bridge!* I prayed desperately. Then I was back on the pavement. (A new bridge is now being built because of the many accidents that have occurred there.)

We were in Kamloops by 4:00 p.m. We attended church the

next day and enjoyed dinner with the person who is head of the clinical laboratory of a nearby hospital.

Gene was so conscientious about the entire undertaking. He was not beyond prodding his mother onward to be sure that every detail fell into place. He used his Bordon's Media Guide to call ahead so the media could meet us as I rode by. Even road repair crews began to recognize us. Sometimes I'd ask them about the condition of the road ahead.

On Monday we crossed the Columbia River and arrived in Revelstoke, the center for all-year recreational activity in the Rogers Pass region. In order to beat the heat and the traffic, I planned to get on the road an hour before breakfast the next day.

Crossing Rogers Pass wasn't as bad as I had expected, although I did put my bike on the rack and walk the last 2.2 miles. In fact, I enjoyed the chance to walk for a while. I remembered Philippians 4:13: "I can do all things through Christ which strengtheneth me," and made up my own rhythm, chanting "which strengthens me" over and over as I walked and rode.

By 5:00 I'd ridden through six tunnels. My dim headlight didn't diminish the darkness very much. I was always thankful when I reached the end of each tunnel. We were traveling one of Canada's most scenic routes, crossing mountains and canyons with densely wooded slopes. The roads were good and the weather sunny and nippy. Outside Golden the roads became narrow, steep, and winding. We pulled in by a fast, turbulent river for the night. Gene, who loves to swim in cold water, went for an icy dip.

Yoho National Park lies just west of the Great Divide and Banff National Park. As I rode along I saw five mountain goats walking across a narrow ledge on a sheer cliff. At Kicking Horse Pass, which is 300 meters higher than Rogers Pass, I walked four-and-a-half miles to the summit, swinging my arms and enjoying the rest from riding the bike. Lake Louise was only two-and-a-half miles away, and we wanted to see it before nightfall. We got permission to park by a large motel near the main road for the night. I felt thankful for making 40 miles that day.

The melting water from Victoria Glacier, from which Lake

Louise springs, carries silt and rock dust that gives the lake its distinctive colors. We arrived at sunset and enjoyed one of the most magnificent views in the world as the colors of the sunset and the towering mountains behind the lake reflected on the water's surface. We rested there on Saturday, thankful we could stay for a whole day. We took our breakfast with us and ate by the lake. Later we hiked around the lake and up to the Tea House, where we were even closer to the waterfalls of snow cascading down the majestic mountain in front of us. Six miles up and back was quite a hike for someone trying to be off the road for the day!

I made excellent time on our way to Banff. At one point I passed a herd of elk standing near the road. Such encounters were a thrill! Banff didn't look anything like I remembered, but of course I hadn't been there in a long time. Townhouses, business establishments, motels, stores, and tourists filled the bustling city. Gone was the silence of the hills. Gene lost me in Banff and almost panicked. He finally found me in front of the Banff Hotel, stalking an elk.

HYPOTHERMIA!

In 1988 I had wanted to celebrate my 70th birthday by swimming across the Okanagan Lake, instead of cycling across on the world's longest swinging bridge. But it had been too cold and too late in the season. Now, because of a cold, damp summer it was still cold, even though it was July. It didn't look too promising for a swim across the lake, but I still wanted to try.

John Fakaro of Aqua Sports graciously loaned me a wet suit that, unfortunately, fit so tightly across my chest it was difficult for me to breathe. Gene suggested that I water ski across the lake to my starting point on the other side. But I hadn't been on skis for a long time and used a lot of energy trying to get up. So we went back to the swimming idea. However, by the time I started swimming I was already shaking and feeling weak.

Distance swimming is not a problem for me, and it was only a mile to the other shore, but I had trouble synchronizing my strokes and breathing rhythmically in the snug wet suit. It wasn't long before I realized this was not going to be the day to swim the lake. Barry McDivitt, a news reporter, pulled me into the boat. I lay on the bottom feeling weak and shivery. By the time we reached the dock I was shivering violently and had a fast pulse and respiration. I felt faint and sick every time I tried to raise my head. Barry and Al Coen, the cameraman, wanted to take me to the hospital. As a nurse, I knew I could monitor my progress, but if I didn't get any better I would need help. Hypothermia can be very dangerous.

After the girl at the boat dock wrapped me in blankets with a hot water bottle I finally began to rally. "Gene, there's no way that I'm going to be able to talk to the media now," I told my son. "If you can get me a cellular phone I'll try talking to them lying down."

In moments Gene was back with the phone. He got the interviewers on the line, put the receiver to my ear, and I did my best to answer their questions. I still couldn't raise my head without feeling faint. I was forgetting details, such as dates, that ordinarily were no problem, a common symptom of hypothermia. After six phone interviews, I said, "No more for now."

After an hour I was finally able to get up. One hypothermia experience was enough.

It would have been easy to leave this episode of "failure" out of my story. But I know it's only when we stop trying and give up that a dream becomes a failure. Even if I'm 90 the next time I have an opportunity to swim Okanagan Lake, I plan to try!

Before we left Kelowna we visited my old family farm in the country. Everything had changed so much I had no idea which road to take. With the help of local people along the way we finally found it. I looked out over the 27 acres where I had played with my brothers and sisters. Things had changed on the farm, of course, but the weeping willow trees, thatched porch, and the same old kitchen brought back many wonderful memories.

CALGARY AND BEYOND

July was almost over, and each new day presented a challenge.

One night we stopped at an old, weather-beaten farmhouse about 18 miles from Calgary to ask permission to park for the night. The woman invited us to park by the house and hook up. She told us her husband had passed away and she lived alone, one of that rare breed who is unafraid to live alone on the prairie.

Before she went into town the next morning she said, "The door will be open; just go in and help yourself if you need anything."

We met people like this woman all across Canada.

One morning I completed 50 miles before breakfast. Sometimes I continued to ride in the evenings after supper. One day I covered 114 miles. Many days I was pedaling 60 to 80 miles. We were near Webb when we stopped at Neil and Lou Cammes' ranch for the night. At times ranchers talked about the hardships and unpredictability of sudden storms, drought, or hail, but for the most part they were upbeat, accepting the bad years with the good.

The days began to pass swiftly. One week of August had flown by already. I welcomed my day of rest each week because it meant no more interviews, no worry about the weather, no cares for 24 hours.

On August 8 I pedaled 94.96 miles; on August 9, 84.18 miles. I stopped at the Saskatchewan welcome center to tell them how much I had enjoyed my ride through their province. When I entered the Manitoba welcome center, the Bamford family rushed up to greet me. They had seen me on television and were very excited about meeting me on the road. Many people said they were following our story in the paper or on TV and radio. Sometimes we had the opportunity to see the newscasts that featured our story.

In two days we would be in Winnipeg!

ESCORTED INTO WINNIPEG

I am not superstitious, but I was glad Friday, August 13, started with good weather and that everything seemed to be in place. Gene arranged for a police escort to meet me 10 miles outside Winnipeg and escort me to the Winnipeg city hall.

"Gene, the idea of stopping traffic at intersections for 10 miles and keeping all those cyclists together without some mishap worries me," I said. "Why isn't three miles far enough?"

"Don't be concerned, Mom. You know everything will be fine!"

We slept at a truck stop outside Winnipeg the night before. I was to meet the motorcade at a trailer sales lot. While I waited I did a telephone interview with CBW-AM radio. Before we started I talked to the police officers and asked them to drive slowly so we could keep up with them.

"You set the pace," they told me.

Three policemen on motorbikes fanned out across the road in front of the procession, followed by a police car. One police officer rode in front of me, another behind. Numerous other cyclists and a pastor on roller blades showed up to join the parade. We began to move forward.

For the occasion I wore a pink-and-white cycle shirt and black cycling pants. My AROUND THE WORLD banner circled my waist, and my white helmet with blue, streamlined trim completed my outfit. Several of the cyclists with us rode expensive bikes and dressed in outfits to match their bicycles. By comparison, my poor old Schwinn Marada looked a little tired and worn. As we rode along, I enjoyed a visit with the deputy on my left. These fellows looked sharp in their uniforms, created especially for cycle cops.

Keeping an eye on my meter, I set the pace at 13 miles an hour. That sounds slow, but we were moving right along. Several times someone asked us to slow down because some of the riders couldn't keep up. The motorcyclists in front were very efficient, swinging wide at every intersection and blocking traffic from both sides.

Frank McMiller, the daredevil, full-of-life clown pastor, was everywhere at once on those roller blades. What made him the proudest, he said, was that sign around my waist and the fact that he was a part of the world tour.

We arrived at city hall with five minutes to spare. Councilor John Pryatanke, representing Her Worship, Mayor Susan A. Thompson, gave a short speech about my visit to his country. He mentioned my own Canadian heritage and made several other nice remarks. Afterward he presented me with a beautiful pin from the mayor.

I responded with a short speech about the friendly and accommodating Canadians, and how privileged I felt to be riding through their gorgeous country. I then presented a subscription of *Vibrant Life* to the mayor. Before we reached the end of our busy day we held television and radio interviews and were on a talk show. Pastor Frank, who had done most of the planning for this event, escorted us out to the highway at 7:30 Sunday morning to say goodbye. He's a dynamo of energy out to change the world!

Three days later we came upon a sign that told us we were "Crossing Over Into Ontario." Numerous small lakes dotted the wooded terrain. No sooner would I pedal by one, mirroring its surroundings, than another waited just around the corner. Some drivers tooted their horns as they went by, spurring me on with new energy. Gene felt concern about how close semis and cars came to me when they passed me on the narrow roads. We stopped at a sports shop in Kenora to buy a vest that would make me more visible to the fast-moving vehicles. The salesman told us that a cyclist from a senior citizens tour group had been hit and killed by a car when a driver swerved to miss another car.

I had been riding all day on an undivided highway with no shoulder. Suddenly I realized a large bus was coming up fast behind an approaching bus. I had just started down a steep hill and was moving at a good clip. I knew I had to quickly move onto the deep shale beside the road or be hit when one bus passed the other. At the speed I was traveling (and without a seat belt) I could easily roll into the oncoming bus or be at the mercy of the gravel. I pumped the brakes, hoping to decrease my speed, and got a tighter grip on the handle bars. Somehow, I made it onto the gravel just as the bus whizzed past me. Although I swerved a little as the cycle came to a stop, I stayed upright.

The mosquito population increased as we traveled east. Recent heavy rains encouraged larvae from previous years to hatch in ditches and flooded areas. As we approached Dryden, I saw an 18-foot sculpture of a moose, a symbol of the plentiful game in the region. Later in the day, with darkness approaching and after 62 miles of travel, we faced the usual question of where we would stop for the night. We ended up in a forest clearing in woods where bears lived. Gene saw one or two on the trip, but not I.

We were meeting very few cyclists on the road. Two men headed west said they were behind schedule because of bad head winds. We were ahead of schedule by several days and began to consider going all the way through all 10 provinces. Our original schedule called for us to go to Gaspé Bay at the end of the Gaspé Peninsula in Quebec. Revising our plans would mean adding 500 miles if we included New Brunswick, Prince Edward Island, Nova Scotia, and Newfoundland. It would cost around $500 to take the ship to Newfoundland and back. We also faced the possibility of ice and snow. We began to pray earnestly that we might know what to do.

Several times we stopped overnight in clearings by the pipeline. Workers had dug immense ditches, 10 to 15 feet across, in order to lay the pipeline. Now it was completed all the way across Canada, except for the stretch where I was cycling. This was the area where they would hook up the final section. Because of the many high hills it had proved the hardest to complete.

The third week in August we stopped for our rest day. We would reach Thunder Bay on the shores of Lake Superior the next day. In addition to several interviews, we took care of such necessities as changing money, buying groceries, and other items of business that can't be escaped even when one is on the road. My bike also received a thorough checkup. Then we enjoyed the opportunity of attending an Indian festival in the afternoon.

That night we stopped at Sleeping Giant Campground. Nearby campers took us in as though we belonged there. Many of them lived there most of the year, swam in the lake, carried in their water, grew little gardens, and generally enjoyed themselves. Some people even had lighted patios beside their trailers. Everyone wanted to know about our trip, and then shared some of their stories with us. A favorite story concerned a bear.

"A bear came right up here on the patio," one woman said. "I told him to go on and leave; this is my place. He obliged."

It was well past our bedtime when we finally returned to our camper for the night. "If there's any charge from the owner we'll take care of it," someone called after us.

THE GREAT NORTH COUNTRY

My bike jiggled across roads cracked from the winter frosts. Sometimes the bike jiggled so badly my eyeballs hurt and my teeth would have fallen out if they weren't part of me. Often my wheels took me to the middle of the road where the highway was a little smoother.

We had to make a decision immediately about revising our travel plans. We would arrive in Nipigon soon, where the road forked. Should we go north on highway 11, or south on highway 17? We chose the Great North Country! Truckers had warned me of the danger of not being seen by semis coming down off the top of the hills.

Just below the junction in Red Rock we enjoyed a stop at a combination ice-cream stand/tavern. Al, a retired bib-overall type with graying hair, played the old, slightly tinny, piano. What he lacked in polish he more than made up for with the music he got out of that piano. His fingers rolled over the keys like waves moving out to sea.

Trapper Monk stopped by while we were there. His long red beard and thick, white-tinged hair sticking out from under his billed cap quickly caught our eye. He called himself the "caretaker of nature." Trapper returned a short time later with his lady friend and her child—and a basket of fresh vegetables from their garden.

So many lakes mirrored the morning light. Such beauty, such silence! I traveled downhill quite a bit now, and the traffic began to thin out. The semis must be taking the southern route. We passed huge Nipigon Lake, where the Royal Windsor Lodge nestled in the trees at the shoreline. Royalty has visited the lodge, and many vacationers from Thunder Bay used to spend the weekends at the lake. But things have changed. Gas and travel have become expensive, and more and more of the cabins remained empty.

I experienced another close call on the road. A semi, moving fast, began to blow his horn frantically—not once, but repeatedly. I swerved onto the gravel, my heart pounding, as he whizzed by. The iron door of some kind of immense iron cage on the back of the truck was wildly swinging open and shut. I shudder to think what would have happened had I not left the road immediately.

At times the weather changed overnight. One day I rode through 92°F. weather; the next day the temperature might drop into the 50s. One day I needed to take extra clothing off; the next day I found myself wishing I had more on. The nights were usually cold.

We were getting closer to civilization now. Two TV interviews, one radio interview, and two newspaper interviews one day meant we traveled 30 miles less than the day before. Time limitations kept us from accepting all the invitations we received. A cycling podiatrist invited us to dinner, but we felt we couldn't take the time. We began to meet more and more French Canadians. They were hospitable and interested in our cause. Sometimes we couldn't understand each other, but we were grateful for the opportunity to get to know them better.

The last day of August I pedaled 14 miles before breakfast. We had made it through Cochrane and were starting to head south. The mosquitoes had taken over everywhere, it seemed, and we had to take cover from dusk on.

The first day of September turned out to be one of my worst—what I call a "character-building" day. The wind, cracked pavement, pipeline traffic, and semis roaring by challenged my cycling skills. Dump trucks on their way to dump dirt from the pipeline scattered loose dirt along the highway. Then the wind and traffic whipped the loose dirt into a frenzy. As evening approached the going finally got easier. I still covered 58 miles that day.

One afternoon I spotted our van ahead, parked on the right shoulder with the bumper flat on the gravel. The right back wheel appeared to be close to toppling over the bank.

"Don't worry, Mom," Gene calmly assured me. "I'll get it out."

He said he had backed up slowly to get a little farther off the road and hit an area where water had gutted out a big piece of the bank. The wheel was now in the hole up to the axle. Gene got the jack out and quickly raised up the right side of the camper. As the wheel came up, stones were wedged into the hole.

A young couple stopped to offer assistance, and the boards in their truck proved to be very helpful. When the tire was finally even with the road, Gene pulled the camper forward and we were free! A little closer to the bank could have been disastrous.

We stopped east of Pembroke one evening, where the swallows congregate each July before starting their autumn migration to South America. We were getting close to Ottawa, which meant we would be back on the media circuit again.

HONORED IN CANADA'S CAPITAL

After biking 32 miles to Capitol Hill I stopped, wondering how I would ever find my way through the traffic. An older gentleman offered his assistance. "I'll go with you and show you how to get there on the bike path that goes all the way into Ottawa." He got his bike, and we were on our way into town. I stared in amazement at the number of joggers, walkers, and cyclists who were out on the path during the noon hour. We rode past lakes, parks, and a river. My kind helper then returned home soon after we arrived at Parliament Hill.

I had the opportunity to speak briefly with the mayor and do media interviews, overwhelmed by the coverage given to my mission. That night we slept in a place overlooking the city and the dazzling lights on top of Parliament Hill. Ottawa is a charming place, steeped in elegance and grace, the epitome of a dignified and beautiful national capital.

Two days later we rode into Montréal. This city also had a path for bikes. On the road I met Richard Kerr, a handsome young man who lived in the area and offered his help. "I'll go with you on the cycle path into town. You might have trouble finding the right path to take at times." Richard's dog accompanied him, sometimes riding in a cart behind the bicycle, and sometimes running along beside the path. I couldn't have found my way without Richard.

The largest television station in Montréal interviewed us and covered our story. The interviewer rode in the camper with Gene as I biked along the road. Somehow they got the pictures they wanted.

That same evening I faced one of the most challenging experiences in my life. It was getting dark, and I needed to be on an alternate route on the other side of the city where the bridge had a walkway across it. I had no idea how to find the bridge, or how far away it might be, and I couldn't keep up with Gene in the heavy traffic.

Then I came to the St. Lawrence River. A mile-long bridge stretched high above the river. Six lanes of cars, semis, and buses roared by in the evening rush hour. It would be suicide to go on the bridge. Gene had already started across in the support van. I stopped close to the cement divider at the side of the entrance and hopped over to talk to some men on the other side. They were getting ready to close two lanes of traffic at 8:00 to make repairs on the bridge. One of them ran over and guided Gene back to where I waited.

"Is there a walk past that wall that goes across the bridge?" I asked several French workmen.

"No, there is no possible way that anyone can ride a bicycle or walk across this bridge. It is just not done, ever. You must go across the city to the alternate route."

"It's already dark and the alternate route is far away. Is there no way you can help me?" I pleaded.

They huddled together again to discuss the matter in French. Finally, one of the men spoke to me in English. "When we shut down two of the lanes to repair the bridge, the police will be here to help direct the traffic into the other four lanes. At that time we can give you a ride across."

"But I must get there by myself!" I protested, showing them my AROUND THE WORLD banner.

They went into another huddle. The minutes ticked away. The evening traffic filled all six lanes on the other side of the divider. *God, You know what to do,* I prayed. *Please help me.*

One of the men spoke again. "Our foreman has gone to get the traffic truck with the bright arrow on top to direct traffic over to the next lane and away from where you are riding. You will ride in front of this yellow pickup. Do not worry; the flashing arrow on top will direct the traffic away from you. Here he comes now."

I promised to ride as fast as I could. The driver of the truck didn't speak English and I wasn't sure if he'd understood what I said, but we started across the bridge. My heart beat faster than it had since the bandits chased me in Nepal. Gene had gone across the bridge ahead of me. There were metal dividers about every 30 feet all the way across the bridge. Each time we crossed one I lifted myself off the seat to avoid the jolt. On and on we went, until I wondered if we would ever get to the other side. My guide stayed right behind my back wheel. If I slipped and fell he might run over me. And what about the cars coming behind him? Would they have time to stop before hitting him?

I knew that once I got to the other side I needed to turn right and meet Gene on a street below the bridge. But I wasn't sure whether the turn was at the end of the bridge or farther on. I must not make a mistake. Then I made a sharp right turn and was out of the traffic. And there was Gene, petrified with fear, standing beside the support van. The traffic truck followed me, pulling in ahead of Gene. I jumped off my bike and gave my French Canadian guide a big bear hug. We couldn't understand each other's words, but we both knew that without him I would still be on the other side of the river.

Why was I so determined to cross that bridge on my own? It was only one mile out of 12,000 I had covered altogether. No one would ever need to know I had ridden in the truck and continued my bicycle journey on the other side of the river. But I would know, and my son would know.

We made between 70 and 80 miles most days, and it looked like we would realize our goal. Three more days and we would be in Quebec City. I was riding on a full-size, smooth shoulder, and felt as light as a feather riding on a cloud. I decided that if the Quebec provincial police stopped me I would ask them to let me stay on the main road. I had been on the velvet strip for several hours when here they came behind me—two handsome officers, well-groomed, and ready for business.

"Can you speak French?" one of them asked me.

"No, sir, I'm sorry. I studied in high school for two years but didn't work hard enough at it."

The other officer spoke this time."You are not allowed on this freeway."

"I feel much safer here and the road is so smooth. And I don't have to worry about the traffic."

"Not even Parliament could give you permission." He was not smiling.

I decided to make one more plea. "My son is back there working with the media. If he loses me it could take a long time to get back together."

It was no use. I could not change their minds.

"Just go on to the next off-ramp and wait there for him."

We visited for a bit, parted friends, and I obeyed the law.

I was getting thinner by the day. Eating every four hours slowed me down too much, so I went back to eating every five hours. That gave me more energy and clearer thinking. I ate a few raisins if my blood sugar dropped in the middle of the morning, and soon I felt the power return.

When we reached Quebec City, we stopped by the old bridge in the main part of the city, near the Parliament buildings. Then we rode in the van across town to the police station to see if we could get permission for me to ride on the Trans-Canada. We enjoyed a delightful visit with the chief inspector, who spoke better English than the others and was eager to practice his knowledge. The answer remained the same, however. "Continue on Highway 132. The scenery is beautiful, and it is quiet through the countryside."

The Parliament buildings in Quebec City are old and, in my opinion, not as impressive as the buildings in Ottawa, Canada's capital. We enjoyed walking through the historical monuments. Across the way, inside high walls, stood the old city of Quebec, where one could go and relive the past.

More media coverage, and then we were on Alternate 132, riding into the countryside. Although the road was sometimes parallel to Trans-Canada, more often it wound through the countryside. I had to admit that the ride through the farmlands was more restful than riding with the 18-wheelers.

We spent the next day down by the St. Lawrence River. The temperature had dropped into the 40s. Gene enjoyed a long walk on the beach, then sat out on the rocks and read for hours, while I enjoyed a good rest. In the afternoon we visited the large cathedral in Joli. Built in 1777, the cathedral's stained-glass windows tell the whole story of Passion Week. The temperature had plunged to 25°F. Would we make it to St. John's, Newfoundland, before winter set in?

More and more people began recognizing me as I rode along. They would see us on television, spot the RV on the highway, and put two and two together. There were really no other through bikers on the road, so travelers had no trouble deciding who that lonely figure out there was.

PRIME MINISTER-TO-BE

We got onto the Trans-Canada again in Rivière du Loup, still in Ontario, but headed for New Brunswick, passing through farmlands and wooded areas. Because we were ahead of schedule, we turned south instead of east. Much of the road was two lanes, so I stayed on it most of the way. No more flashing red lights pulled me over! That night we were very sleepy, but happy to be on our way. Tomorrow we would leave Quebec.

We were out with the dawn the next morning and crossed into New Brunswick about 2:00 p.m. I enjoyed excellent roads and a shoulder most of the way and, sometimes, a tail wind. My legs coped pretty well with the stress of the upward slope of the road. I was beginning to feel a sense of urgency, though, as I rode through the fall colors because we were two-thirds of the way through the month of September.

We decided to go to Grand Falls to see if we could meet Liberal Jean Chretien, who was running for the office of prime minister. He was to speak at a high school there. When all the speeches were over, Mr. Chretien graciously stood between Gene and me, with one arm around each of us, so we could have a photograph taken of the three of us together.

Soon after daybreak the next morning I started pedaling in a dense fog. I couldn't see more than 20 feet in front of me and, frankly, it was very scary. I came to another bridge and stopped. If a car came behind me, or one car passed another, they wouldn't see me until it was too late to slow down. Gene was somewhere behind me on the road, so he couldn't follow me across. But even if he could, cars traveling through the fog probably wouldn't be able to see our slow-moving white camper.

"God, take care of me," I breathed, and started across the bridge, moving as fast as I dared in the fog. I had come through dangerous experiences on other bridges, and God brought me safely across this one.

We stopped in White Cove that night and stayed in the yard of the MacLean brothers. These middle-aged bachelors, well-known in the community, had developed an interesting conversational style. While they both talked at once, they talked slow enough so that one could separate the sounds. There they stood by their immaculate little house the next morning watching us drive away, both still talking at once.

If we were going to cross over to Newfoundland we had to either borrow $500 to get there and back on the steamer, or ask God to provide it in His own way. Gene checked on the Maritime Atlantic ships and spoke to contacts in Newfoundland. He seemed pleased with the results.

Sunday night we arrived just in time to catch the 6:30 ferry to Prince Edward Island. It was hard to judge exactly how long it would take to meet these ferries, and it seemed we always arrived just as they prepared to pull out to sea. The next day would be my 75th birthday.

The next morning I was on my way to Charlottetown from the Borden Pier. I spent a great deal of time with the media and didn't cover many miles that day. I spoke to the students at the Colonel Grey High School in Charlottetown, who gave me a warm reception. When the principal introduced me, the mayor, who is also a teacher, said he hadn't had time to get me anything, but could he have a bear hug? Then everyone sang "Happy Birthday" as the principal and I walked out.

Gene was somewhere behind me when I came to the bridge leading out of town. I stayed close to the guardrail, walking and pushing my cycle, to keep from being knocked off my feet by a strong wind, and slowly made my way to the other side. As I progressed, it was calmer. I realized I was riding over the top of the hills with less effort now and, of course, I got to rest and go faster down the other side.

We needed to catch the boat at the south end of the island. Cars were already coming off the ferry, and it was getting dark. I couldn't see very well and kept dodging potholes. Then I saw Gene ahead of me. Once more we made it onto the deck moments before the gangplank went up.

Gene was in contact with Newfoundland, organizing everything for the grand finale. Kelly's Mountain would be the big hurdle. I told Gene to tell me when I got to it, but he decided I would do better climbing it if I didn't know I was already near the top. He encouraged me by coming up behind me, yelling to me in his booming voice that I would soon be at the top. I am happy to say that I made it all the way, although I probably would have walked more of the way if I had known where I was!

And then we arrived in North Sydney, Nova Scotia. I had reached the other side of the continent! I hugged the first person I met, who happened to be the service station attendant. We went down to the North Sydney Pier, our departure point for Newfoundland, and parked in the church parking lot. In the night I awakened to strange sounds outside the camper. I opened the blind a little and saw a tall, thin teenager in a bill cap standing beside my bike.

"What are you doing out there?" I yelled at him. He took off so quickly you'd think a bear was in hot pursuit.

We went to church the next day. We would leave that evening to sail to Newfoundland. And the $500 fare? Gene had written to Marine Atlantic, telling them we were anxious to visit the province, and that I would like to ride around the "rock," as people called Newfoundland. Marine Atlantic had agreed to pay our way over and back, including stateroom and food. Praise the Lord, from whom all blessings flow!

When Gene took the bike off the rack in the parking lot, he

discovered that the outside peddle and the seat clamp were missing. I wanted to start riding the next morning as soon as the boat landed. But there was nothing really we could do. I told Gene to wait and see what God would do in our behalf. He called a couple places to see if we could bring the bike. Carl Baudreau and his mechanic Gus drove 20 miles to Carl's bike shop to help us. Carl put on two pedals, better than the ones I had, some new toe clips, and a new clamp to hold the seat. Gus noticed the right brake wasn't working properly and needed to be replaced. I knew I'd be going down some steep hills, and if the brake didn't work properly I might end up with more than a missing pedal. Gus checked the bike all over and oiled it, and then my faithful companion was ready for the challenge of the "rock."

"What do I owe you?" I asked.

"Twenty dollars will be fine."

As we were loading the bike onto the van, Carl came outside and insisted we take back the money as his contribution to our cause.

If I hadn't called out the window to that boy the night before, he could have had the bike off the rack and stripped down before morning.

THE ROCK—NEWFOUNDLAND

October was definitely here. Canadian geese honked their plaintive warning that it was time to bring in the final harvest. Would we beat the clock? Eric McDonald, who was in charge of the harbor at night, visited us in the RV before we started our trip to Newfoundland.

"I am very happy to be able to honor you by sending you across to Newfoundland on Marine Atlantic," he said. "Canada thanks you for coming to our country with such high ideals and a desire to have us work together to stay healthy and reduce the cost of health care. It is an honor to present these tickets to you."

When we landed in Channel-Port aux Basques, I walked up the steep hill from the harbor to the highway. The bike operated better than ever. I hadn't been on the road long when I came to an area where the winds blasted off the coast with demon-like fury, buffeting me from one side to the other. At one point the wind picked up the bike, with me on it, and dropped us out on the traffic lane! Another blast of wind hit me in the chest with such force that I was stopped in my tracks, still upright, but not going anywhere. Black clouds gathered overhead and it started to rain. I was chilled to the bone when I arrived at Petra Canada. By then the gale had changed to a tail wind, moving me along at great speed. I hated to stop, but it was getting dark and enough is enough. I had covered 60 miles and gotten as far as Crabbes River.

"Mom, did you know you just came through Canada's Wreck City, the windiest place in Canada?" Gene asked.

Wreck City earned its name because of all the wrecks that happened there. Sometimes the winds through the city reached a gale force of 150 miles an hour. At times, semis had been turned over and people had abandoned their cars and crawled over to buildings to get out of the evil blast. The news reported that 50- to 60-mile-an-hour winds had blown through Wreck City that day. I felt thankful not to be one of the statistics.

It was October 4. I had to be in St. Johns, on the other side of the island, by the 12th. The beauty and silence of open space soothed my body and spirit as I biked over the roller-coaster coast. Great boulders raised their rough-cut sculptures into the clear, blue sky. No smog or contaminated lakes disrupted the serenity of the area.

I hurried toward Corner Brook. We planned to meet some schoolchildren who would ride into town with me. By the time we arrived, reporters from CBC and two other stations, plus the newspaper, had congregated at a downtown store. Church folk and other well-wishers came to meet us.

Winter was beginning to breathe down our necks. The cold air mixed with drizzly rain was bearable, though unpleasant. Gene located some insulated gloves for me to wear, which helped a great deal. It would be a tight schedule to make it to St. John's, meet our obligations there, then catch the ship back the next day. We were supposed to take the church service the next day at Benton, but

Gene called the pastor to say we couldn't make it.

"My daughter lives in Gobbles," the pastor said. "She will pick you up and take you back to wherever you are parked."

So we spoke in their quaint, little white church and enjoyed a tasty dinner before returning to our camper.

We hadn't reached Gobbles yet, and Gobbles was 75 miles away from St. John's. The final ceremony was scheduled to take place at 1:00 p.m. on Tuesday at the "0" marker in downtown St. John's. Usually every day had more good weather than bad, but Sunday was one of those days that was all bad. The cold wind and rain blew at me sideways so that I could barely see or move forward.

"Gene, please drive me ahead 20 miles or so, then I'll ride back to where I left off, taking advantage of a tailwind." (There were no rules as to which direction I had to go, just so I covered the miles.)

So Gene drove me ahead, dropped me off, and headed back to where we had started to wait for my arrival. The bike and I flew down the road. It was warmer, I could see where I was going, and the wind helped to push me along. I grabbed quick meals and continued to ride. We were still on the road at 9:45 that night. It was dangerous because Gene had to follow behind me, shining his headlights so that I could see ahead of me.

The closer we got to the finish line the next day the more horns we heard, urging me on. I thanked God for a day with no rain, good roads, and good visibility. We kept going until 8:00 p.m., with Gene lighting the way as he'd done the night before.

When we stopped at a little business center, the hotel manager came out. "I kept Terry Fox here, and made a ramp for Rick Hanson to roll in his wheelchair. You can stay here too if you wish," he told us.

Before we could go to sleep, however, we needed to discuss what to do. I still had more than 50 miles to travel to reach the center of St. John's City. We must arrive by 1:00 the next day to meet the mayor, the press, and the president of the Seventh-day Adventist Newfoundland Conference. What about the children waiting to escort me the final eight miles into town? I'd have to put in more miles now if we were going to meet the deadline. But how could I ride in the dark on a road without a shoulder? We didn't have time to come back and do this section later. Finally, I made a decision.

"Gene, I'll go on and you come behind me. Flash your lights every time a car is coming and I'll get off into the gravel."

The whole thing frightens me now as I think about the dangers of the road at night. The cool air was invigorating, and I wouldn't let my mind dwell on anything else but the task before me. I made excellent time in the light traffic. The darkness finally faded away. I don't know when I've been happier to see the light in the eastern sky.

Then I ran into another difficulty. The temperature had dropped to two degrees above freezing. My nose was numb and my gloves were not insulated adequately to keep my fingers from losing feeling. I needed both hands to change gears frequently and to use the brake handles. Several times I had to stop and go inside the camper to thaw out and get a glass of hot water. Gene put hot water in my bottle every time I stopped.

By 9:30 I began to lose my strength. I knew I was burning a lot of calories, and I certainly didn't want anything more to do with hypothermia. I realized my blood sugar was dropping, so I went inside the camper and started gulping down leftover mush with raisins. One of the teachers who had arranged the meeting with the students came looking for us. I wonder what he thought my chances were when he saw me slumped in that chair swallowing mush.

"We forgot to tell you that the last 20 miles into the city are worse than anywhere else on the island for hills," he said.

Just what I needed to hear! Gene urged me out the door. I knew it was humanly impossible for me to get to the Trans-Canada "0" marker on time and in one piece on my own. So I prayed as I rode, and asked God for a special favor.

I had spent a total of one year on the road and had ridden more than 12,000 miles, often alone, without any human help to encourage me or with whom to discuss the next move. I wouldn't have been out there at all if I hadn't been sure that God and the heavenly angels were my constant companions. My prayer changed to "With these hills, I know I don't have enough time to get to where the children and the police escort are before 12:15 so that we can get into town by 1:15. You will have to take over. Thank You."

Gene had gone on ahead to give the media my approximate location on the road so they could plan their schedule and not have to wait for me. I rode on, going through the motions. From somewhere I received the strength to climb the hills, thinking that surely each one would be the last. Then my heart would sink when I looked ahead and yet another hill loomed before me. Finally, though, I rode over the top of the last hill and let the bicycle fly down the other side.

I arrived 15 minutes late at the first appointment place and had just enough time to give a few directions, rearrange my layers of clothing, and line up behind the motorcade. We arrived at our destination 10 minutes early. No more heavy traffic, no holes in the road, no more fear of crashing into the bike next to me. The trek was over!

The conference president appeared right on time. I had a little time to visit with him before the mayor arrived. The mayor gave a short speech and handed me a lovely pin and a large picture book of St. John's. All the media covered the event. Someone brought some water from the Atlantic shoreline and poured it over my foot as I stood before an immense sign designating the place where the Trans-Canada had begun. We talked to some of the media back home, and Gene contacted the U.S. national news, Associated Press, Reuters News Service, Canada Press, and ABC and CBS national radio news.

The church arranged a reception for us that evening, complete with a lovely dinner and after-dinner speeches and the gift of a book on Newfoundland. I knew they had gone to a lot of work to make it a special occasion for us.

That night we drove down and stayed on the dock so that we'd be ready to sail in the morning. Once more we received guest tickets, meals, and a stateroom for the 14-hour trip back to the mainland. With tickets in hand and hearts singing we boarded the *David Smallwood* and once more headed out to sea.

Thank you, Canada, for allowing me to come back home and accomplish an adventure that I needed to realize. I have received more than I've ever given, and the tie with the country of my birth has grown too strong with memories and love too sweet to ever be broken.

My faith has grown deeper and my love for my heavenly Father stronger as He and His angels guided me one day at a time until I crossed the finish line.

Epilogue: As we go to press, more than two busy years have elapsed since the end of my journey. Both my husband, Gene (who helped with the mail drops), and my brother Arthur (who told me to keep my feet straight on the pedals) passed away before my global trek was completed. In 1995 I closed the books for the last time as a volunteer assistant professor at Andrews University in Berrien Springs, Michigan. God has continued to protect and guide me, just as He did on the road.

My son, Gene, and I moved to Washington State to a home at the base of a mountain overlooking the North Cascades. I have a big garden, where I grow every known vegetable and flowers galore. In winter we cross-country ski six days a week to keep in shape. In summer we backpack and hike a new trail into the mountains every weekend. We'd really like to hike the Pacific Crest Trail that runs from Mexico to the Canadian border. (We're looking for a llama to pack our gear.)

We've held cooking schools and have just received the go-ahead for a weekly radio program on health-related issues. And who knows what else we'll get into! How thankful I am that I have good health and can do about whatever I want to.

Feel the Difference
Vibrant Life Makes

Vibrant Life lets you know how to feel your best. Get life-changing advice on nutrition and fitness. Discover simple ways to avoid disease. Enjoy wholesome, delicious recipes.

If you want to experience more strength, more energy, and more peace of mind, subscribe to *Vibrant Life,* the one health magazine that recognizes the connection between faith in God and your well-being.

Credit card orders: 1-800-765-6955.

☐ Please send me one year (six issues) of *Vibrant Life* for only US$9.97.* I save 33 percent off the cover price of US$15.00.

Your Name _____

Address _____

City _____

State, Zip _____

Please add US$5.10 per subscription for addresses outside the U.S.A. Mail with check or money order to: *Vibrant Life,* P.O. Box 1119, Hagerstown, MD 21741.

* Price subject to change.   651-03-0